S0-BXW-754

DON'T LOSE YOUR PATIENTS!

DON'T LOSE YOUR PATIENTS!

RESPONDING TO CLIENTS WHO WANT TO QUIT TREATMENT

Herbert S. Strean

JASON ARONSON INC.
Northvale, New Jersey
London

Production Editor: Robert D. Hack

This book was set in 12 pt. Fairfield Light by Alpha Graphics in Pittsfield, NH.

Copyright © 1998 by Jason Aronson Inc.

10 9 8 7 6 5 4 3 2 1

All rights reserved. No part of this book may be used or reproduced in any manner whatsoever without written permission from Jason Aronson Inc. except in the case of brief quotations in reviews for inclusion in a magazine, newspaper, or broadcast.

Library of Congress Cataloging-in-Publication Data
Strean, Herbert S.
    Don't lose your patients : responding to clients who want to quit treatment / by Herbert S. Strean.
       p. cm.
    Includes bibliographical references and index.
    ISBN 0-7657-0171-5
    1. Psychotherapist and patient.   2. Patient satisfaction.
  3. Dropouts—Psychology. I. Title.
    [DNLM: 1. Psychotherapy—methods. 2. Patient Dropouts—
psychology. 3. Professional-Patient Relations. 4. Patient
Satisfaction. WM 420 5914d 1998]
RC480.5.S7239 1998
616.89'14—dc21
DNLM/DLC
For Library of Congress   98-17725

Printed in the United States of America on acid-free paper. For information and catalog write to Jason Aronson Inc., 230 Livingston Street, Northvale, New Jersey 07647. Or visit our website: http://www.aronson.com

To my patients
(including those who terminated prematurely)—
teachers all!

Contents

INTRODUCTION

When I reflect on my forty-five years spent practicing psychotherapy, I realize that the times I have been the most anxious were when I sensed correctly, or felt incorrectly, that a patient was getting ready to leave treatment prematurely. Moreover, the times I have been the saddest were when patients had definitely made up their minds to depart from me before I wanted them to go.

For a number of years I tended to believe my own separation anxiety and fears of abandonment were stronger than those of most of my colleagues—hence, I assumed that I became more overwhelmed and helpless than they were when confronted with the possibility of a patient quitting treatment. Yet when I began to supervise, teach, and participate in peer supervision, I learned that I was not such a special case! I discovered that virtually all clinicians, whether engaged in private practice or employed in a social agency, have a strong desire to keep their patients in treatment until termination becomes a mutually agreed-upon decision based on their therapeutic progress. In fact, when patients threaten to leave therapy prematurely, most practitioners refer to this event as "losing" patients because they are deeply concerned about the *loss* of income, the *loss* of personal self-esteem, and the *loss* of professional status.

Those of us who supervise practitioners soon learn that many clinicians, if not most, choose to discuss with us mainly those patients who are threatening to leave therapy and/or those whom the therapist thinks might do so. Furthermore, most supervisors also realize quite early in their supervisory work that practitioners are very eager to learn what to say and what not to say to their patients so that they will want to sustain their treatment contacts with the therapist.

Despite the close to universal interest among mental health practitioners in avoiding patient dropout, the literature on the subject is very sparse. Apparently, clinicians have found it difficult to put into print their deep concerns about losing money, losing self-esteem, and losing professional status. Often, we mental health professionals need to hang onto our omnipotent defenses, and not acknowledge openly blows to our narcissism, threats to our wishes to feel competent, and signs that we don't know it all!

It is of interest that the handful of professional books and articles on the dynamics of why patients leave therapy prematurely (for example, Chessick 1971, Strean 1986, Wolman 1972) focus mainly on the patient's "poor motivation," "unresolved transferences and resistances," "negative therapeutic reactions," or "intense narcissism." Very few books and articles focus on the therapist's contributions to premature termination, the mismatch between patient and therapist, or what practitioners might have said or done or not said or done to avoid the premature termination. I recall that when I was a doctoral student in the 1960s I was told to memorize the "fact" that patient dropout occurs when there is insufficient motivation, capacity, or opportunity in the patient (Ripple et al. 1964). The therapist's motivation, therapeutic capacities, or learning opportunities didn't seem to account for much.

One of the main reasons we can now consider the therapist's contribution to the premature termination of treatment is that psychotherapy in the 1990s is conceptualized very differently from the way it was heretofore. Patient and therapist are now considered equal partners who constantly influence each other and they are both "more human than otherwise" (Sullivan 1953). The days of the wise, stable doctor ministering to the unwise, unstable patient no longer exist. Therapists are busily exploring their unconscious motivations for practicing psychotherapy (Sussman 1992) and are trying to face their countertransference actions and reactions on a daily basis (Consolini 1997, Schafer 1995).

Although Freud discovered "the countertransference" in 1910, as Racker (1972) pointed out, it took many decades before countertransference became a subject discussed frequently in the literature. Racker claimed that clinicians did not pursue the scientific investigation of countertransference because their unresolved neurotic conflicts prevented them from recognizing unresolved countertransferences. He asserted that clinicians have a strong desire to feel complete and perfect, and dread feeling incomplete and imperfect.

As Abend (1989) has stated, "Freud's original idea that countertransference means unconscious interference with [a therapist's] ability to understand patients has been broadened during the past forty years: current usage often includes all of the emotional reactions at work" (p. 374). Slakter (1987) has referred to countertransference as "all those reactions of [the therapist] to the patient that may help or hinder treatment" (p. 3).

Because countertransference and transference are now considered as constants in therapeutic interaction, it is now *au courant* to view premature termination as a contribution of both therapy partners, much as a dynamically oriented clinician would view two marital partners ending their marriage through divorce as a joint responsibility.

This book is an attempt to focus sharply on the therapist's contribution to therapeutic divorces. While I strongly believe that both patient and therapist influence this outcome, in this book I want to concentrate mainly on the therapist's contributions. The reason for this is now obvious: the therapist's role in his or her "losing patients" has been very much neglected in the professional literature.

About ten years ago I was asked to give a talk entitled "Why Therapists Lose Clients" (Strean 1986) to a group of therapists. It was the best-attended talk I have ever given, inasmuch as the topic aroused all that interest. Since that time I have been gathering data on this very provocative and most stimulating phenomenon. I have been studying when and how my colleagues and I have failed to listen to our patients and talked too much instead; how we have hastened to answer our patients' questions when we would have been better off exploring their motives for asking; how we prevented our patients from voicing anger, sexual feelings, and other affects because they threatened us too much; how we directly and indirectly acted out our own contempt toward patients; how we failed to appreciate the meaning of our patients' transference reactions and other means of resisting our help.

What has been of much interest to me as I have been studying why patients leave therapists is how the patient's unresolved problems often are mirror images of the therapist's. What used to be a horrendous realization is now commonplace—the patient's mental health and ego functioning can often be superior to the therapist's.

These countertransference problems will be alluded to frequently throughout this text as they emerge at different stages of therapy. In addition, I want to demonstrate the impact of other unresolved countertransference problems, such as the therapist's fear of her own compassion (Bernstein 1972) and her fear of other primitive affects (Maroda 1994). A common countertransference issue that will be explored is the therapist's desire to "rescue" the patient and therefore become therapeutically overambitious. What I have also observed consistently during this past decade as I have been intensively researching why patients leave therapists is how one countertransference of the clinician's can lead to others. For example, if the patient's pathology reminds the therapist of her own, she may wish to deny the intensity and pervasiveness of the patient's struggles and then misdiagnose the patient. Then, when a patient, for example, suffers from a borderline personality, he may be incorrectly diagnosed as a neurotic and then given an inappropriate treatment experience.

In directly working with and supervising the work with patients who stir up therapeutic impasses (Kantrowitz 1993), I have slowly come to appreciate the value of sharing counter-transference reactions with the patient at crucial times (Maroda 1994). For example, when I have told a rebellious and provocative patient that he is inducing in me angry and/ or hurt feelings, a more mutually rewarding therapeutic inter-action is likely to ensue. Disclosing to patients at pertinent times my feelings of helplessness, impotence, and/or strength and pleasure has often helped overcome an impasse and restored a therapeutic relationship that was about to dissolve. I intend to demonstrate this form of therapeutic interven-tion a few times in the following pages.

Although I strongly endorse the notion that the aware-ness by the therapist of her countertransference is a *sine qua non* in preserving the therapeutic relationship, I believe that the critical guiding factor for the therapist is the patient. If one listens carefully to the patient, he emerges as the best psychotherapy consultant available (Langs 1976, Maroda 1994, Searles 1975, Strean 1970).

In order to appreciate the struggles and vulnerabilities, as well as the wishes, hopes, loves, and hates of our patients that very much influence how they respond to our help and therefore determine in many ways whether they remain in treatment, we have to be in tune with "the child" in them and "the child" within ourselves. Racker (1968) championed this proposition when he said: "We must begin . . . to accept more fully the fact that we are still children and neurotics even when we are adults and analysts" (p. 130).

In this book I would like to focus on patients' plans, threats, and wishes to quit treatment *at different stages* of their treatment. In the early chapters, I will attempt to demonstrate through case illustrations and theoretical discussions how and why patients want to quit treatment during or immediately after their initial telephone request, during or immediately after their first interview with the practitioner, during the honeymoon phase of treatment, and during the first treatment crisis. Later chapters will deal with threats and wishes to leave therapy during the middle to later stages of treatment. In addition to reviewing the unique dynamics of different patients who want to quit treatment at different stages of it, I also want to discuss the therapist's contributions to compounding the patient's resistances to treatment, focusing on the therapist's countertransference reactions that lead to inappropriate therapeutic interventions.

My attempt in this book is to present to the practitioner not only appropriate therapeutic interventions which can sustain the therapy, but to offer a perspective of treatment that combines careful listening, a nonjudgmental approach, and a realization that the therapist, like the patient, " is more human than otherwise" (Sullivan 1953). I am also of the opinion that because the therapist's individual psychology constantly determines her posture, as Renik (1993) has clearly demonstrated, "awareness of countertransference is always retrospective, preceded by countertransference enactment" (p. 556). Just as no patient who is in the middle of a transference reaction is consciously aware of his distortion—does not say, for example, "I am now making you my seductive mother"—the same may be said of the practitioner and her countertransference responses. It is only after the countertransference enactment that the therapist may become aware of the nature of her personal involvement.

All of the case illustrations in this book deal with real patients who have been patients of mine or patients of supervisees, students, or colleagues. Identifying data have been altered in order to preserve confidentiality.

No book is the sole creation of one person. Therefore I would like to thank the many individuals who have made it a reality. First and foremost, I would like to thank my wife, who has compassionately listened to my professional dilemmas and struggles for over four decades and in addition has competently edited and typed my books and articles with dedication and devotion. Our sons, Dr. Richard Strean and Dr. Billy Strean, continue to be my favorite critics—constantly helping me to better conceptualize psychotherapeutic practice. To my many colleagues, supervisees, and students who have shared with me their thoughts and questions, including many of the case illustrations in this book, my profound gratitude. And, to my friends at Jason Aronson, Inc., my deep thanks for their consistent cooperation, particularly Dr. Michael Moskowitz, Norma Pomerantz, Bob Hack, and Judith Cohen. Finally, this book could not have been written without the help of the many patients who have entrusted me with their care—to them, my abiding love and gratitude for their direct and indirect counsel.

CHAPTER ONE

A Good Therapist Is a Good Telephone Operator

The first contact between therapist and patient is usually over the phone. Despite the ubiquity of this event, the dynamics of the first encounter are rarely discussed at clinical conferences or in the professional literature. Because there are few dynamic principles on which practitioners agree regarding the first phone contact, clinicians' responses to it tend to be idiosyncratic and quite subjective. Some therapists have lengthy discussions with prospective patients, eliciting many facts, a great deal of history, and other data; others have a very brief conversation and try to schedule a consultation interview as soon as possible.

In my supervisory work and in my discussions with colleagues, I have learned that many cases are lost during or right after the first phone conversation. A large number of clinicians tend to minimize not only the importance of this event for patient and therapist, but also can underestimate how very anxious, ambivalent, and apprehensive most prospective patients are when they finally make a decision to ask for professional help. Moreover, therapists frequently are not fully aware of how they themselves feel and appear over the phone when talking to prospective patients.

The decision to pick up the phone and ask a therapist for a consultation is rarely, if ever, a spontaneous act for most individuals. Many patients, after they have been in treatment for several months, report having started to call a therapist for the first time and then putting the phone down even before hearing the therapist's voice. This same scenario can be repeated many times by them. Particularly in American culture, where autonomy is championed (Kardiner 1945) and dependency is demeaned, individuals often consider it a sign of weakness and failure when they reveal their need for professional help with their psychological and interpersonal problems.

Although few prospective patients directly state over the telephone how frightened they feel and how dubious they are about receiving therapeutic help, the way they conduct themselves over the phone often tells us how agitated they are. A barrage of questions about how therapy works, how long it takes, what the practitioner's qualifications are, what the therapist's theoretical predilections may be, and how much she charges, usually reflect how uncertain the prospective patient feels about undertaking treatment. If the therapist is not sensitive to the fact that requests for information usually are a reflection of the applicant's anxiety and therefore cannot be answered factually but must be explored instead, the prospective patient will not feel very well understood by the therapist.

I recall when I was a beginning practitioner, I received a phone call from a prospective patient who asked, "Can you tell me the times you can *not* see me?" Unaware that her query revealed an unconscious wish *not* to meet with me, I answered her question directly and told her when I was occupied. The applicant never arrived for an appointment. At least one of the reasons for this was that I did not show her that I understood that a big part of her did not want to begin therapy with me.

Clinicians soon realize that, despite the pain and anguish that prospective patients endure, they have enormous fears about altering the status quo. These fears or *resistances* to being helped are manifested from the first phone call right through termination of treatment.

Many clinicians, especially beginners, are so determined to get a prospective patient into therapy, particularly if they are in private practice, that in their eagerness and enthusiasm they fail to relate to the applicant's resistances (Strean 1990) and, instead, doggedly attempt to set up a consultation. This rarely brings the consciously desired result.

Another situation that I flubbed as a beginning practitioner was when a man called me and made a most revealing slip over the phone. He said, "I'm desperately in *need of trouble!*" He wanted to say he was "desperately in need of help," but instead revealed his unconscious wish to stay in trouble. Eager to get him into my office, I bypassed his wish to maintain the status quo, and he never did become a patient.

I believe that because many clinicians are so eager to get applicants to become their patients and very fearful of losing this opportunity, they provide too much reassurance over the phone, answer too many questions, and then can cause an intimidated, ambivalent prospective patient to feel too overwhelmingly anxious and very unprepared to begin therapy.

The sensitive, empathetic clinician shows in her attitude over the phone that the caller does not have to make a commitment to arrange an appointment pronto. She is not in a rush to bypass resistances by answering questions readily, nor is she tempted to provide a lot of reassurance, which usually looks suspicious. Instead she is interested in sounding receptive, and, without getting involved in a long dialogue over the phone, suggests to the prospective patient that the caller *might consider* meeting her face to face so that questions, concerns, and doubts, which always exist, may be discussed in a consultation. I have found that most prospective patients respond positively to this approach, and if they insist on having their demands·gratified over the phone, in all likelihood they are not really ready to begin psychotherapy.

Too frequently therapists impose conditions for therapy over the phone that only serve in most cases to alienate the prospective patient. To tell an apprehensive applicant that he should consider twice a week therapy when he wants once a week or less only compounds resistances. When the applicant wants to come alone to the consultation to discuss a marital problem, but the therapist says that he should bring his wife with him, only induces feelings of anger, rejection, and alienation. Prospective patients make many outlandish requests—desires to meet a mate, receive sexual stimulation, opportunities for sensitivity groups, changes to their religion or gender, or many other fantastic demands. The sensitive clinician does *not* say over the phone that she does *not* render the service requested, but invites the prospective patient into her office to discuss the request further, so that the prospective patient can feel better understood eventually. A maxim from social work that is pertinent to all of psychotherapeutic practice is "Begin where the client is" (Hamilton

1951). This means that regardless of the client's request over the phone (or later), the request is empathized with and studied, rather than rejected or gratified. When the applicant observes that the therapist is trying to understand, he usually feels more willing to become a patient.

Inasmuch as the vast majority of prospective patients are individuals having difficulty liking themselves, they are very ready to feel misunderstood or rejected. Consequently, the more the therapist asks questions over the phone, the more possibility there is for the applicant to find something offensive. If clinicians want the applicant to become a patient and appear in their offices, they should listen to their prospective patients' requests patiently, suggest that questions about schedule, fee, the therapist's qualifications, and so forth, could be discussed in more detail face to face, *if the prospective patient would like this*, and then see how the applicant responds to this invitation. If the prospective patient responds with doubt or uncertainty, the therapist can empathetically show that she understands that the prospective patient may have some doubts about meeting her. Then, feeling understood, most prospective patients do make an appointment. In those cases where they don't, prospective patients can be warmly told that they may wish to call back at a later date. Often this stance does eventually bring them back.

In this chapter, I want to focus sharply on those issues that usually pose difficulty for prospective patients and prospective therapists that emerge during the first telephone contact. As I mentioned in the introduction, the case illustrations that we will be discussing are real examples of real telephone contacts. Names and identifying data are disguised.

DEALING WITH THE REQUEST

There are some prospective patients who can pick up the phone and tell the practitioner that they would like to meet with her to have an interview as soon as possible. When the clinician offers a time, place, and date for an appointment, she then has her first opportunity to ascertain how the prospective patient feels about therapy. Well-motivated individuals, those who may be compliant and/or cooperative, and those who feel they are in crisis frequently accept whatever appointment time is offered, and do come in for an interview. This of course does not mean that resistances to therapy will be absent in the first interview or the last.

I have found that if the applicant is ready to accept the appointment as presented, I then can give him instructions to get to my office and tell him that I am looking forward to meeting him on the designated date. I ask no further questions or make any further remarks. I have plenty of time to hear about the prospective patient's situation when he comes to my office.

If the prospective patient has difficulty adapting to the times offered by the practitioner, this is usually a sign of his anxiety. I have found that after a couple of appointment times are rejected by the prospective patient, it is not productive to offer more. Rather, it is more helpful to the applicant to make some empathetic remark about his difficulty in arranging an appointment time.

Andrew, a man in his early thirties, called Ms. B., a private practitioner, for a consultation because he had "difficulty establishing relationships with women." Although Ms. B. offered Andrew several possible appointment times, he had many reasons why none of them was convenient. Insensitive to his anxiety and not dealing with his resistance, Ms. B. gave Andrew a date and time that he thought he "might be able to make." Andrew did not show up for his appointment nor did he call to cancel. Andrew and Ms. B. never met each other.

When an applicant for psychotherapy finds it difficult to work out an agreement about an appointment time, invariably we know that a big part of him does not want an appointment. It's too scary! In the above case of Andrew, we could anticipate his reluctance to make an appointment. He had "difficulty establishing relationships with women." Consequently, he was not going to establish a relationship with Ms. B. easily. Ms. B. did not realize that sooner or later all patients usually relate to the therapist the same way they relate to others. A transference begins with the first phone call (Strean 1990).

> When Andrew called another therapist three weeks later, he again had difficulty finding a proposed time and date convenient for him. However this therapist, Ms. C., handled the situation differently. After Andrew turned down three proposed appointments, Ms. C. said warmly, "It's awfully difficult coming to a therapist. Most people feel uncomfortable right before they have their first appointment. Would you like to wait a while before you make an appointment?"
>
> Hearing Ms. C.'s nonthreatening and accepting remarks, Andrew felt understood and did make an appointment,

which he kept. He stayed in therapy with Ms. C. for over two years.

One of the most common errors that clinicians make during the initial phone interview is to experience the applicant's request too literally. Many prospective patients hear from others and/or tell themselves that they need something like sex therapy, or group therapy, or family therapy, psychoanalysis, or possibly marital counseling. What they say they need may or may not turn out to be an accurate assessment. However, all too often therapists are ready to tell these patients what they need is what the practitioner specializes in—turning a deaf ear to what the patients say they need.

Many cases are lost over the phone when the clinician does not "begin where the client is." Professional staff from social agencies and mental health centers often are inclined to tell applicants over the phone that they do not work with particular modalities and thus alienate prospective patients right away. It is perfectly ethical and is good therapy to accept whatever the patient is interested in doing and suggest to him to come in for an appointment and discuss it in further detail.

After Daisy, a single woman in her thirties, had called three therapists requesting "a sexual cohort" and was either told she needed psychotherapy or was rejected altogether, her fourth telephone call yielded more satisfying results. Dr. E., when he heard what transpired in the previous telephone calls, tried to be more related to Daisy's request. He told her that he was interested in discussing her need for a sexual cohort in more detail. Feeling accepted, she made an appointment and kept it.

When Daisy met Dr. E. she told him of severe sexual inhibitions and an intense dislike of sexual intercourse. As Dr. E. tried to understand the roots of Daisy's difficulties, she gradually moved into intensive psychotherapy. Her desire for a sexual cohort quickly dissipated.

Although many therapists respond too literally to their applicants' requests and alienate them as we have already suggested, other therapists respond with too much eagerness to their patients' requests. Over the phone, therapists often tell prospective patients that they are experts in the modality requested and are very sure they can be of much assistance. Although they are not always consciously aware of it, prospective patients feel manipulated when they are promised a great gift after barely being acquainted with the therapist.

Frank was a senior citizen who called an intake worker of a social agency in order "to expand my social relationships inasmuch as they are currently too superficial." Ms. G., the intake worker, told Frank that she was sure she could help him. Her agency had many groups for senior citizens and there were many people who would be glad to meet him. Although Frank seemed to accept the idea of coming for an intake interview, he never arrived at the appointed time.

When another worker at the same agency, Mr. H., called Frank a couple of weeks later to try to find out what happened to him, his statements were very revealing and instruc-

tive. Averred Frank, "That lady sounded too interested in
having me. I kind of felt I was with an insecure salesperson.
She boasted of her product so much, I thought she was protesting too much."

RESPONDING TO THE
REFERRAL PARTY'S PRESCRIPTIONS

Most individuals who seek out mental health practitioners
are recommended to do so by friends, family, colleagues, or
other professionals. Usually these referral parties have their
own diagnoses and treatment plans for the prospective patient and frequently have convinced him of their validity.
When the prospective patient calls for help, he may be so
well indoctrinated that he requests a special type of therapy
for a very specific condition.

Although it may be that the referral party knows what
he's talking about, he may not. Very often, because the applicant is ambivalent about help, he can unconsciously arrange
for the referral party and the prospective therapist to get into
an argument. By externalizing his ambivalence about receiving therapeutic help, the prospective patient can rational-
ize away his need for help, feeling that those who are supposed to know are really all mixed up. Therefore, in his mind
therapy and therapists become unreliable.

Isabella, a woman in her forties, was referred by her physician to Mr. J., a therapist in private practice. Isabella
had severe migraine headaches, gastrointestinal difficul-

ties, as well as phobias, compulsions, and other neurotic problems.

Over the phone, Isabella told Mr. J. that her physician felt she was suffering from severe anxiety and needed intensive therapy. Eager to reassure Isabella that her condition was not so awful, Mr. J. told her that she probably could be helped by having weekly therapy. To his surprise, Isabella told Mr. J., "If my doctor says one thing and you say another, I don't know what to believe. I'll have to think this over." Isabella never did make an appointment with Mr. J.

Following her phone call with Mr. J., a few days later Isabella called Ms. K., a psychologist in private practice. On hearing about the disagreement between Isabella's physician and Mr. J., Ms. K. tried something else. She told herself that inasmuch as Isabella had a closer relationship with her physician than she did with Mr. J., it would be a good idea to reinforce the physician's diagnosis and treatment plan.

When Ms. K. told Isabella that she knew her physician, thought well of him, and tended to endorse his prescriptions, she, too, received a response that surprised her. Said Isabella, "If you and Mr. J. in the same field can't agree, what am I supposed to do?" Attempts to get her to make an appointment were futile.

The case of Isabella, who was very ambivalent about help, teaches us that most of the time it is unwise to take any stand over the phone. Because most prospective patients are ambivalent about requesting help, when the clinician reinforces one side of the ambivalence, the prospective patient is inclined to take the other. If either Mr. J. or Ms. K.

in the above vignette had told Isabella in a neutral but friendly manner that it may be a good idea to come in and discuss the doctor's recommendation together, the results may have been different.

In some research I did over twenty years ago on the dynamics of referring a patient for psychotherapy (Strean 1976), I learned that all referrals contain an unconscious message emanating from the referral source to the recipient of the referral. I said:

> Referrals may be expressions of love, hate, or ambivalence; they may be manifestations of rivalry and competition or defenses against these drives. Inevitably they reveal something about the psychodynamics of the referring party and his transference to the person to whom he is referring the prospective patient, and to the prospective patient himself. A resistance to the understanding of the personal and interpersonal forces operating in the referral transaction may lead to patient dropout and to the compounding of patient resistance and [therapeutic] counterresistance. [p. 131]

As I have studied the referral process further and discussed it frequently with colleagues, I have concluded that referral sources can be categorized. There are some referral sources who are almost always dependable—the individuals they refer almost always become patients. There are other sources whose referrals hardly ever show up. Finally, mixed results emanate from referral sources who are ambivalent toward us.

Just as children often express the unconscious feelings of their parents, prospective patients frequently reflect the unconscious affects of those who have referred them. It is a good idea to find out over the phone who referred the applicant to us and remind ourselves of the referral source's track record with us.

> A therapist in private practice, Dr. L., reported to his colleagues in peer supervision that a former supervisor of his referred prospective patients to him frequently. The only trouble was most of the individuals that the former supervisor recommended never called and those who did never showed up.
>
> When Dr. L. discussed this situation with his former supervisor, he learned that the supervisor envied Dr. L.'s success as a practitioner, resented that he did not need the supervisor any more, and unconsciously sabotaged the referral process.

Dr. Murray Sherman (1966), over thirty years ago in *Psychoanalysis in America: Historical Perspectives,* said something about the dynamics of the referral process that is still pertinent:

> Over a period of time, a particular therapist may develop a particular type of practice built upon his past successes, failures, and sources of referral. The referral process itself would likely be most resistant of all to scientific appraisal, but there is doubtless a subtle social interchange that occurs but receives little attention in terms of the psychological and even unconscious significance involved. A determined researcher would find this a most rewarding field of investigation. [p. 20]

DEALING WITH THE PRACTITIONER'S QUALIFICATIONS

By far, the most frequent question asked by a prospective patient over the telephone is, "Could you tell me about your qualifications?" What practitioners often fail to appreciate is the obvious—when the prospective patient makes this query *he is questioning the therapist's qualifications*. He wonders whether the therapist can or will help him.

When a prospective patient is wondering about the possibility of being helped, and therefore is suspicious of the helping process, the most wonderful professional qualifications are not going to reduce his anxiety. Rather, this applicant needs to be shown in an empathetic manner that perhaps he is not sure whether the practitioner can help him.

What clinicians often overlook when they are on the phone with someone applying for help is that most prospective patients have been told about the practitioner's qualifications prior to the phone call. Furthermore, the referral source has usually recommended a therapist of whom he has spoken positively. I have made an axiom of psychotherapeutic practice for myself: when a prospective patient questions my qualifications, I try to explore his doubts about me. If I don't do this, he probably won't become a patient.

> Mary, a 40-year-old married woman, was referred to Ms. N. for marriage counseling. Over the phone, Mary asked Ms. N., "Do you know anything about bad marriages and how to fix them?" Ms. N. responded to Mary's question by telling her of her long experience working with all sorts of conflicted

marriages and that she was an expert in individual therapy, conjoint marital therapy, and family therapy. Sounding impressed, Mary nonetheless said that she wasn't ready to make an appointment and never did with Ms. N.

One of the pitfalls in stating one's excellent qualifications is that the prospective patient can feel intimidated by a professional who has so much stature. When the applicant for psychotherapy calls a prospective therapist, at a time when he is feeling low himself, he is looking for compassion (Lewin 1996) and empathy, not somebody who flaunts her superiority. Hearing about outstanding qualifications often induces in the applicant the feeling of being a second-class citizen. If one feels like a second-class citizen, a means of coping with this ignoble position is to attempt, albeit unconsciously, to make the therapist feel vulnerable. This can be done by rejecting the therapist, as Mary did to Ms. N.

> Mary in the above case illustration called Ms. O. a week later. Again, she asked Ms. O. if she knew anything about marriages and how to fix them. Ms. O. replied, "Usually when people ask me about my qualifications, they have some questions about me. Would you like to come in and see for yourself how we do when we talk about your marriage?" Mary, after a moment's silence, said, "I like your approach. You're not a braggart. The last professional I spoke to tried to impress me with her great qualifications. I concluded she was desperately trying to get new patients!" Mary made an appointment with Ms. O. and stayed in treatment for several years.

Sometimes a prospective patient is very insistent about knowing about the professional's background and doesn't take "no" for an answer. Although the applicant may appear intimidating, this is no cause for the therapist to capitulate. I have learned that the prospective patient who is insistent, provocative, and intimidating, although belligerent at first, welcomes a firm response primarily because the therapist who does not capitulate is considered somebody one can respect.

Peter, a man in his forties, sought help from a mental health center in his local community. On the phone he told the intake worker that he had a lot of sexual problems but he wasn't sure that the intake worker, Mr. Q., was able to handle "a tough case" like his. When Peter learned that Mr. Q. would be his therapist if he came to the mental health center, he asked Mr. Q. over the phone, "Are you familiar with the latest sexual therapy techniques?" Mr. Q. said, "I get the impression you are not confident that I have the stuff to help you." Brusquely, Peter retorted, "I'm *not* confident that you have it. That's why I'm asking you a question." Then he inquired again, "I want to know, do you have the knowledge to help me?" Mr. Q. responded, "I could tell you about some of my knowledge but I think it would help you more if we met and you could see for yourself if you were helped." After a silence, Peter said, "I'll think it over and call you back if I decide to come in."

Peter called Mr. Q. to make an appointment two days later. In the initial consultation, he told Mr. Q., "When I saw that you didn't get ruffled by me, I knew you knew your stuff."

THE USE OF MODALITY

As we have already suggested, many prospective patients, influenced by others and/or by their own biases, often suggest over the phone what kind of therapy they need. In our current mental health scene there are literally dozens of therapeutic modalities for sale and dozens of theoretical orientations being utilized. Prospective patients often have some strong convictions about what they need or don't need. But what happens when the prospective patient says over the phone to a Freudian clinician who specializes in intensive individual therapy, "The one thing I don't want is a Freudian who does that long-term stuff!"? Or what if the prospective patient wants conjoint marital therapy and that is the practitioner's first love? Should she share that information over the phone?

I believe that the two most common errors that mental health professionals make on the phone are stating that what the prospective patient desires they can't provide or pointing out that what is requested is exactly what is available. The reason these stances turn out to be errors is that, as already implied, what people feel they want, they may not need. Somebody wanting short-term treatment may need many sessions. A man who wants to acquire some new sexual techniques may need to talk about his fear of and hostility to women. A woman who wants individual treatment may get more from a group.

Because requests that contain the prospective patient's preferred modality need to be studied in one or more interviews, I believe it is always more helpful to the prospective patient not to have the therapist's theoretical predilections revealed over the phone. First of all, it is the rare clinician who can be sure about what a patient needs before meeting him. She has to study his request thoroughly and get to know more about his history, current modus vivendi, and a host of other factors before formulating a treatment plan. Secondly, I have found that most prospective patients feel much better understood and more supported when the therapist says, "I think it might be a good idea for us to get to know each other better so that we can decide together what's best for you. At this point I don't think I can be sure. How about coming to my office and talking it over with me?"

WHO SHOULD COME TO
THE FIRST INTERVIEW?

Many cases are lost over the phone because the therapist is too inclined to state dogmatically who should come for the initial interview. If she is a specialist in long-term individual treatment, the therapist might too quickly tell a woman who is fighting daily with her husband, and desperately wants marriage counseling, to come alone to see her. Or the therapist who is a specialist in family therapy or conjoint marital counseling may fail to recognize that the individual who is speaking to her over the phone may very much want a confidential one-to-one interview.

Although all clinicians are entitled to have their preferred methods of working—with individuals, couples, families, or small groups—in order to avoid losing patients over the phone, they have to be able to begin where the client is.

As the therapist listens to the phone applicant describe his problems and situational difficulties, she often can infer correctly if the caller wants and needs a one-to-one interview. For example, if the caller talks exclusively about himself, the chances are quite high that he needs a private interview. On the other hand, if the prospective patient constantly refers to his wife and/or his child, the chances are greater that he may need a conjoint or family interview.

In most cases, the individual who can answer the question, "Who should come to the first interview?" with the greatest degree of accuracy is the caller himself (Maroda 1994). Furthermore, if the individual making the phone call is consulted on this issue, diagnostic material of pertinence often becomes more available.

> Rhoda, a woman in her forties, called Dr. S. and told him over the telephone of her very conflicted marriage of ten years. She mentioned that she and her husband, Sam, had continual arguments "about so many things—money, sex, the children," that her married life seemed very much like a war.
>
> As Dr. S. listened carefully to Rhoda, he was quite sure that she and Sam needed conjoint marital therapy and that this would be Rhoda's preference. However, when Dr. S. asked Rhoda if she would like to come for an interview with Sam, or alone, she strongly responded, "I must see you alone. There are a lot of things I don't want Sam to hear about. Seeing you alone is a must! Is that okay with you?"

Dr. S. assured Rhoda that he could see her in a one-to-one interview, and did so. At this interview, Rhoda revealed she was having an extramarital affair that she did not want to discuss with Sam, who was not privy to this information.

Sometimes clinicians who feel they do not have any expertise in working within a particular therapeutic modality are reluctant to have a consultation that involves an interview outside their area of expertise. Yet, if the prospective client is the best judge, it is helpful to adapt to his preferences and see what happens in the consultation interview.

When Tom, a 30-year-old man, requested that he and his wife be seen in conjoint treatment, the therapist, Ms. U., although working exclusively in one-to-one therapy, agreed to Tom's request. As Tom and his wife felt very much individualized and empathized with, at the end of the consultation, they both requested individual therapy with Ms. U., which worked quite well.

What happened with Tom and his wife in the above illustration does not always occur, that is, the patient chooses the modality at which the therapist is an expert. Sometimes it is necessary for the therapist, after a face-to-face consultation, to refer the prospective patient to a colleague who has expertise in a modality in which the therapist does not. Usually a prospective patient can accept a referral with more confidence after he has had a favorable experience with a therapist in consultation. The important point I wish to stress is that telephone applicants for therapy are more apt to accept the idea of a consultation if they are consulted on the matter of who should come for the initial interview. If their ideas are respected, they are more inclined to remain in treatment with the therapist or accept referral to a colleague.

THE INVOLUNTARY PATIENT

If it is difficult for individuals who voluntarily seek psychotherapy to reveal themselves to a stranger, imagine how vexing it is for an involuntary patient to call up a therapist! Yet many prospective patients have been commanded to see a therapist by a boss who threatens to fire him, a spouse who threatens to divorce him, or a fiancee who will not marry him unless he undergoes treatment. Although the criticized spouse or lover, troubled student, or adjudicated criminal may initially welcome treatment rather than face the alternative of divorce, being thrown out of school, or being sent to prison, he usually resents that he is being forced into treatment (Strean 1991). Because the involuntary patient usually resents the idea of treatment but often cannot tell anybody this, the skillful clinician knows that, unless the prospective patient's resentment is faced and discharged, therapy will have a limited effect or none at all.

As we suggested earlier, one of the essential tasks of the therapist on the phone is to determine who referred the prospective patient and how he is responding to the referral. By confronting this task we will usually learn if we have an involuntary caller. If so, we have to be able to demonstrate to him over the phone that we are compassionate and can empathize with his dilemma. Showing compassion for the difficult position he is in often animates the phone conversation (Lewin 1996).

> A college student of 19, Victor, phoned Dr. W., a private practitioner, and told him that he "must have therapy." When Dr. W. inquired why Victor "must" the latter told him that he would be thrown out of college if he didn't get into therapy right away. On Dr. W.'s asking Victor how it felt to be forced into therapy, Victor replied, "It's okay." When Dr. W. quizzically said, "Really!" Victor said, "I have no choice."
>
> Dr. W., sensing how trapped Victor felt, compassionately stated, "It's damn tough to be forced into something—particularly something like therapy, which can go on for a while." Sensing that Dr. W. was a possible ally, Victor said, "You seem to understand how much of a jam I'm in. I'd like to meet you."

Much of Victor's therapy with Dr. W. involved looking carefully at Victor's readiness to submit to authoritative pronouncements without realizing how much he resented "capitulating." Had Dr. W. not related over the phone to the predicament that Victor was in, the therapy would not have gotten off to the excellent start that it did.

I have found that therapy never works when the patient feels under legal, moral, or psychological coercion. If an empathetic, non-authoritarian attitude is shown to the patient from the first phone call on through the treatment, therapy has a much better chance of succeeding.

CALLS ON BEHALF OF A
PROSPECTIVE PATIENT

A difficult phone call for the therapist to cope with is from the individual who is calling on behalf of a prospective patient, instead of the patient himself. Often a wife phones a therapist to arrange treatment for her husband, or a parent may do the same for a child. Often therapists are recipients of phone calls from sons and daughters who want to make appointments for their parents. I have received many calls from men and women who want to make appointments for their friends.

Often, when the therapist asks the caller to have his spouse, child, parent, or friend call the practitioner, the person never calls. Frequently when an appointment is made by one person for another, the appointment is broken by the person for whom it was made.

When one person calls a therapist for another, the person calling is often, albeit unconsciously, asking for help for himself. Most of the time the spouse, parent, child, or friend who calls for someone else does not feel free to ask directly for therapy and finds it easier to ask for help for someone else. However, if the caller's unconscious wish is interpreted over the phone and he is told he is indirectly asking for treatment for himself, the caller will probably deny it. Therefore, to respect the caller's latent wish for help and concomitantly respond to his resistance to therapy, the sensitive therapist will ask the person making the call to come in and discuss his child's, spouse's, or friend's problem. Many parents, spouses, and friends welcome the possibility of an appointment for such purposes, and if empathetically responded to by the therapist, they often become patients in their own right.

> Yolanda, a single woman in her thirties, called Dr. Z., a female therapist in private practice, to discuss her friend, Alice. Over the phone, Yolanda told Dr. Z. that Alice was a very insecure person who needed much therapy but found it difficult to ask for it. On being asked by Dr. Z., "What do you suppose is in Alice's way?" after a long pause Yolanda responded, "She can do for others but she can't take care of herself."
>
> Dr. Z. noted to herself that Yolanda's description of Alice as one who does for others but can't help herself might also apply to Yolanda. After all, Yolanda was doing for others by calling up Dr. Z. and asking for her friend to be helped.
>
> When Dr. Z. asked Yolanda how she would feel coming in to see Dr. Z. and discuss Alice some more, Yolanda seemed surprised. She said, "I'm only interested in help for a friend, but . . . if that's what you want, I'll try it."
>
> After Yolanda met with Dr. Z. for two interviews and spent a lot of time talking about Alice, she was able to ask for help for herself. Dr. Z., realizing that Yolanda's statements about Alice were self-descriptions, handled her responses empathically but deliberately.

FEES

Almost as frequent as queries about the practitioner's professional qualifications are questions about the practitioner's fees and fee policies. Many clinicians believe that the phone caller has "a right to know" the fee before making an appointment and do tell him when asked over the phone. I do not subscribe to this point of view, for several reasons. First, many prospective patients may think the fee mentioned over the phone is too high and either turn away from the practitioner or try to bargain with her. When two people, who have never met face-to-face, are in a bargaining situation, they are not likely to resolve it easily and therefore it does not seem to be a good way to begin a relationship. Second, the fee offered over the phone could sound too low to the applicant, and then he may begin to have doubts about working with the practitioner who does not value herself enough. Third, as is true with many of the issues that we have discussed in this chapter, prospective patients and therapists have a better chance to determine what the fee will be after they have had a warm face-to-face interview. Many issues between two people have a better chance to be resolved in the flesh than over the phone.

When a prospective patient asks me over the phone what the fee will be, I tell him that I'd like to determine that with him when we meet. Most prospective patients seem to respond positively to this suggestion and do come in. Like most practitioners, I have a pretty good idea about what I want my fees to be, but I try to keep the fee arrangements flexible. Even if the therapist is adamant about the fee she is going to charge, she is usually much better off discussing it in a face-to-face interview. Very often after a reluctant prospective patient meets the therapist, he is more inclined to accept the fee that is asked.

Bob, a 30-year-old man, called Ms. C. because he needed help so he could "give up my single status." On Ms. C.'s suggesting that he come in and discuss it further, Bob said he would very much like to do that but needed to know Ms. C.'s fee. When Ms. C. told Bob that her fee was $100 a session, Bob said it was too high and did not make an appointment. Despite the fact that Ms. C. said she would be glad to reconsider the fee, Bob remained adamant about not making an appointment.

Two weeks later Bob called Dr. D., a male therapist. When Dr. D. was asked over the phone what his fee was, he told Bob that he would like to determine that with him when they met. Bob came in for an interview, discussed his problems, and shared some of his history. At the end of the interview, Dr. D. said, "My usual fee is $100." Bob willingly accepted.

Money is a highly cathected subject in our culture. Many people's self-esteem is based on how much they are worth financially. Furthermore, how we value other people often depends on their financial assets. That is why the issue of fees needs to be explored sensitively and empathically in the therapeutic situation.

One reason that motivates people to seek psychotherapy is a wish to have a loving relationship with a parental figure. To pay for this opportunity often conjures up associations in the patient's mind that he is visiting a prostitute or someone similar.

Erik, a married man in his forties, phoned Ms. F., a therapist in private practice, because he wanted help for his "shaky marriage." After a mutually pleasant phone conversation, Ms. F. was asked by Erik, "How much do you gals get for this stuff? I know you don't believe in free love!" When Ms. F. told Erik she had the impression that he had some questions and feelings about paying for her help, he replied, "I feel like a fool paying to be serviced."

Money and fees, like most of the issues we have been discussing in this chapter, do not cease to be concerns after the first phone conversation between therapist and patient. Money and fees are of concern to both parties throughout the entire treatment process.

HOW MUCH DOES THE THERAPIST DISCLOSE ABOUT HERSELF?

Throughout this chapter one of the central themes has been how much the therapist discloses about herself. Does she tell the prospective patient what her professional credentials are? Does she discuss her fee policy? Does she reveal her preferred therapeutic modalities or her theoretical predilections?

Self-disclosure has become a very much discussed and very controversial subject among contemporary therapists (Goldstein 1997, Raines 1996). While I believe that there are times when it can help the patient and advance the therapy if a therapist shares some aspects of her life and/or selected countertransference reactions with the patient, I am wary of doing so at the beginning of treatment, either during the initial phone call or in the first interviews. The reasons for this are several. As we have already suggested, when we don't know the patient well, we can't be certain how he will react to our disclosures. Further, questions about the therapist's life, as we have indicated, are usually an expression of the prospective patient's doubts and anxieties about therapy and the therapist, and therefore should be explored as to their meaning rather than immediately answered.

One of the problems in answering personal questions at the beginning of treatment is that the patient then has "the right to have encores." Why shouldn't patients whose questions about the therapist are initially answered assume the right to have all questions answered throughout the whole treatment process? By answering personal questions at the beginning of treatment, we can make it more difficult for the patient to absorb the inevitable frustrations that will come later in treatment.

It has been my consistent observation that therapists who answer personal questions at the beginning of treatment are frequently doing so to ward off the patient's anger or wish to reject the therapist. I have also found that when therapists do not need to protect themselves this way and can listen to the patient's disappointment, resentment, and criticism of the therapist when his questions are explored and not answered, as hostility is discharged in what begins to look like a safer environment, mistrust recedes and a therapeutic alliance begins.

This issue often becomes salient in the first interview between therapist and patient, to which we now turn in Chapter 2.

CHAPTER TWO

THE FIRST INTERVIEW: THE MOST CRUCIAL ONE

Assuming the phone call between prospective patient and therapist went smoothly, the parties are now ready to meet face to face in their first interview.

It cannot be emphasized enough just how important the first interview is. If the prospective patient and therapist communicate well, and the patient can tell her story and feel she is being listened to with empathy and understanding, the chances are quite good that the patient will continue in treatment. On the other hand, if the patient feels misunderstood, unsupported, imposed upon, or spoken down to, she will probably not want to return for further treatment.

Although few therapists and few patients would disagree with the above, most of the time when patients don't return for further therapy after the first interview their dissatisfactions, fears, and resentments were something they were unaware of, and often the therapist was unaware of exactly what transpired between them. Many clinicians have frequently expressed the following sentiment after the first interview: "I thought we related quite well. I was quite sure I understood her so I was very surprised when I heard she did not want to return."

It has been estimated that as many as one third of the individuals who have an initial interview with a therapist do not return for further help (Strean 1978). Despite this high incidence of failure, there has been limited study of the first interview in psychotherapeutic practice. Yet, as learning theorists have demonstrated, according to the "law of primacy" (Hall and Lindzey 1957), our first experiences with something or somebody tend to be the most influential. We are apt to remember our first day of school better than our tenth, hundredth, or five hundredth. The same applies to our first romance, first sexual experience, or first trauma. Consequently, patients are likely to govern their attitude toward psychotherapy by how they are treated in the first interview.

THE PATIENT'S STRUGGLES

One of the paradoxes that every patient in psychotherapy demonstrates is that despite the suffering she endures daily, manifesting itself in unsatisfying interpersonal relationships, neurotic and psychosomatic symptoms, feelings of low self-esteem, and other maladaptive problems, the patient also wants to cling to the status quo. Clinicians become aware rather early in their careers that all patients, consciously and unconsciously, resist telling the truth about themselves and frequently fight the process of learning the truth about themselves.

By the time an individual seeks therapeutic help she is usually quite desperate (Fine 1982); nonetheless, the prospective patient is frequently ashamed to reveal her childish wishes, self-destructive defenses, and those past and present experiences about which she feels guilty. One of the crucial variables that colors the first interview is that the prospective patient, who often views herself negatively, tends to project her self-image onto the therapist and is ready to be judged negatively. Very often, as the patient approaches the first interview, she tends to ascribe her own punitive superego to the therapist and consequently expects to be demeaned and castigated for her vulnerabilities and imperfections.

One of the reasons that some prospective patients, particularly involuntary patients, enter the first interview with a chip on their shoulder and an axe to grind is that they are convinced they are going to be attacked and demeaned, so they attack first. I remember a man who walked into my office for the first time and before he sat down said, "How can people tell their problems to you? You look as if you are emotionally disturbed!" When I suggested that perhaps he would prefer not to talk to me about his problems, he replied, "No, I'll hang around a bit. Maybe it'll make me feel better to talk to someone who is inferior to me."

When men, women, or children enter a therapist's office for the first time, they are reminded, albeit unconsciously, of feelings and experiences they had with those who were entrusted to listen to their problems and then resolve them. If these caretakers could not be trusted and were either unresponsive, unempathetic, or not genuine, prospective patients will anticipate being treated similarly by the therapist.

Although it is the strong and courageous who seek psychotherapeutic help, most prospective patients tend to feel, at least somewhat, that they are weak and incompetent if they need therapeutic help. That is why many prospective patients are antagonistic toward the therapist. They feel like a second-class citizen next to him.

Inasmuch as those who seek therapeutic help have been told by family, friends, and other professionals to "stop worrying," "leave your wife," "go on a vacation," or "take up a hobby," and these prescriptions haven't yielded much satisfaction, they are wary about receiving some more unsolicited advice that will have little to do with their emotional conflicts.

THE THERAPIST'S STRUGGLES

When a therapist meets a prospective patient he, too, has many anxieties. Although sometimes difficult for him to acknowledge, like his counterpart he also is apprehensive about being found incompetent and/or unlikeable. He, too, is unsure which of his vulnerabilities and limitations will be exposed. Further, he worries about what the prospective patient will present that he won't be able to handle. Inasmuch as clinicians are "wounded healers" (Sussman 1992), they often are concerned about how much healthier their patients are than they.

Because the therapist is probably more anxious in the first interview than he is in many others, he may forget that his prime task in the first interview is to listen. He may be so eager to impress the prospective patient with his expertise that he will ask too many questions and/or make several premature interpretations. He may fail to keep in mind that when the prospective patient talked to others about her problems, she received too much advice, too much false reassurance, and too many other unhelpful remarks.

When therapists can monitor their own anxieties during the first interview, they will adhere to the notion that what relaxes a prospective patient who feels frightened, self-conscious, and vulnerable is a quiet, nonintrusive, and empathetic listener. Listening tends to diminish the prospective patient's tension, builds her self-esteem, and inspires hope. When an individual in distress feels warmly accepted by being carefully listened to, she begins to accept herself with more warmth and the world begins to be a somewhat better place. If the therapist can provide a safe and secure atmosphere, the patient begins to feel similar to a loved child who can get ahead in life under the guidance of a caring parent.

In this chapter, we will review and discuss some of the main reasons why prospective patients drop out of treatment after the first interview. Although there are patients who must defeat the therapist no matter how well intentioned the therapist is, and despite the fact that certain resistances to treatment of the patient are too powerful for any clinician to handle, our concern in this chapter, as it will be throughout most of the book, is on the therapist's role in patient dropout and what can be done about it.

FAILURES IN LISTENING

From the moment an individual begins the therapeutic process, she has feelings, fantasies, and fears about the helping person. These reactions are frequently expressed by the prospective patient skeptical of the therapist's ability to help, and raising questions about the efficacy of therapy.

One of the most serious mistakes that a therapist can make during the initial interview is trying to reassure the prospective patient that the therapy will have a positive outcome. What is often overlooked is that if the patient can talk openly, at length, and in detail about her doubts and uncertainties, with the therapist carefully listening to the patient's words, the patient is more apt to feel understood and supported. On the other hand, if she is frequently reassured, she is less likely to come back for a second interview.

> Adele, a college student in her late teens, came to a college mental health center complaining of depression, poor grades, and a very limited social life. When she told her female therapist that she had never been in therapy before and was not sure how it worked, Adele received a great deal of reassurance from the therapist. Adele was told that she just had to do her job, which was to talk and say everything that came to her mind. If she did, the therapist was sure she could help her. On leaving the therapist's office, Adele said, "I hope it works," but she did not return for a second interview.

It is important for mental health professionals to keep in mind that virtually all prospective patients carry all kinds of distortions about therapy, particularly if they have never been in treatment before. When patients point out that they are not sure how therapy works or what roles befit patient and therapist, they are getting ready to discuss their doubts about therapy and are questioning whether it will help them. The therapist needs to encourage the patient to discuss her doubts, not try to talk her out of them.

> When Adele, in the above example, saw another therapist a couple of weeks after her first experience, she again voiced her indecision about beginning therapy and her doubts about whether it could help her. The male therapist not only told Adele that practically all newcomers to therapy have their doubts about it, but that it would be helpful if she could tell him what she pictured therapy would be like.
>
> Adele very much appreciated the therapist's attitude and went on to tell him that she expected the therapist to tell her what she was "doing wrong" and offer "criticism." The more Adele talked in detail about her distortions of the therapeutic process and the more the therapist carefully listened, the more Adele could eventually see how she was getting ready to make the therapist a punitive superego. As she discussed in more detail her readiness "to be put down," she could recall how this was her experience at home where she was constantly nagged.
>
> Because Adele had a therapist genuinely interested in listening to her doubts about treatment, she could begin to form a therapeutic alliance (Greenson 1967) with him and continue in therapy.

Inasmuch as the 1990s is the decade of managed care and short-term treatment, many mental health professionals are in a hurry to do therapy right away. The work must get done quickly because the treatment process will end in ten or fewer sessions. When the interviewer feels pressured to take a history, establish a definite diagnosis, and create a working alliance—all in one session—he is not in a position to listen with free-floating attention. Rather he will be inclined to interrupt the patient frequently and impose his own needs on the patient.

> John, a 50-year-old man, was seen by a male therapist because he was involved in a very conflicted marriage for a long time. In his first interview John told the therapist that they had twelve interviews to "fix up" his marriage and that "the person from managed care assured" him that it "usually took that amount of time to straighten things out."
>
> Pressured by the edict from managed care, the therapist bombarded John with many questions about his past and present, gave John a diagnostic appraisal of his marriage, and arranged for treatment to begin the next day. John did not return for another interview.

In this day and age of quick fixes and instant gratification, therapists, like everybody else in our society, can be seduced and manipulated by what is the current trend. Many mental health professionals in their wish to be *au courant* with current cultural norms can forget that psychosocial growth, if it is to be effective, takes time. They can overlook the fact that most patients would rather talk freely about their feelings, thoughts, and memories than be asked many questions and rushed into treatment. When the therapist is not in a hurry, the patient has more of an opportunity to think and grow. John, in the case above, told his second therapist that he needed a clinician who "does not bombard me or rush me and make me feel I'm with my controlling wife."

ASKING QUESTIONS

Although the therapist's primary task, particularly during the initial interviews, is to listen, he is also interested in the patient's history, the details of her current situation, and other pertinent data; consequently, he does need to ask some questions.

One of the ways that an attentive listener demonstrates that he has grasped the essential points of the patient's story is through his questions. A question that truly engages the patient will be one that clarifies ambiguities, completes a picture of the patient's situation, draws out more detail on her thinking, and elicits emotional responses (Kadushin 1997).

In order for a question to be considered helpful by the interviewee, she has to experience it as one that, if answered in full, will enhance her in some way. Questions that can be answered with "yes" or "no" do not really help the patient discharge tension, explore her situation more fully, or increase her self-understanding. For example, asking a prospective patient, "Are you happily married?" gives her little opportunity, because of the way the question is phrased, to reflect on her marriage, discharge her complaints, or examine her role in it. However, if the clinician asks, "Could

you tell me about your marriage?" more data will be elic-
ited and a fuller exploration of the patient's marriage may
ensue.

While questions have to be phrased so that they can be
understood—unambiguous and simple enough so that the
patient can remember what is being asked—perhaps more
important than the precise formulation of a question is the
attitude with which it is presented. The patient must feel that
the question evolves from the interviewer's empathy and iden-
tification with her. This helps the interviewee want to talk
freely, communicate more in depth with the clinician, and
really tell her story.

> When Carla came to a family agency to see if she could
> place her mentally retarded daughter in an institution, she
> tended to describe her daughter in intellectual terms,
> focusing on her limitations, vulnerabilities, and pathology.
> After listening to these affectless designations for about
> twenty minutes, the social worker, feeling the absence of
> emotion from Carla, empathically asked, "How is it for
> you living with a youngster who does so little for herself?"
> Within seconds, Carla began to talk about how the child
> was "draining . . . very hard to take . . . and gets me angry
> all of the time."
>
> Carla then went on to voice her anger, despair, and hurt
> for the next twenty minutes. Near the end of her interview,
> Carla said, "You know, before I place Dorothy, I'd better
> talk some more with you about how I feel. I'd hate to place
> Dorothy if it was just out of anger. Let's see if she really needs
> an institution, or if I just want to get rid of her."

FAILURE TO RELATE TO THE PROSPECTIVE PATIENT'S EARLY TRANSFERENCE REACTIONS

One of the greatest contributions of dynamic psychotherapy to the mental health professions is the notion of transference (Freud 1912). Transference is a universal phenomenon that dominates each individual's interpersonal relationships and exists in all of them, personal and professional, formal and informal. Because all of us bring our unique histories, ego functioning, superego mandates, fantasies, and fears into all of our human interactions, nobody perceives anybody without some distortion. In all interpersonal relationships non-rational, subjective factors are present.

If clinicians do not understand how they are being experienced by their patients, they cannot be very helpful to them (Fine 1982, Freud 1912, Strean 1994). All patients respond to their therapists' interventions (verbal and non-verbal) in terms of their transferences. If a patient loves the therapist (for example, sees him as an ideal parental figure), the patient will be inclined to accept most of the therapist's interventions. If the patient hates the therapist (transfers onto him qualities of a hated parent, sibling, or teacher), even the most neutral question by the practitioner will be suspect. Finally, if the patient has mixed feelings toward the therapist (the most common transference), almost all of the therapist's comments and actions will be experienced ambivalently.

Although many transference reactions are quite overt in that the patient can consciously feel love, hate, or ambivalence toward the clinician, and may even point out that the therapist reminds her of a parent, teacher, or sibling, in most instances transference reactions are subtle and covert and have to be inferred. This is particularly true in the first interview.

Although transference reactions are present from the first phone contact and become strengthened as the patient approaches the first interview, the main way for the therapist to decipher them in the first interview (and in later interviews) is to listen carefully to how the patient describes people in her past and present environments. For example, if at different times the patient describes a mother, father, and a teacher as individuals who listened attentively to the patient, then there is a strong possibility that this is the way she is experiencing or expects to experience the person who is interviewing her. On the other hand, if the prospective patient refers to a doctor, minister, and librarian as unhelpful, the chances are quite high that this is what the patient is transferring onto the therapist.

If negative transference reactions are not related to in the first interview, then the patient may act out the angry feelings and drop out of the treatment abruptly.

Frank, in his early twenties, was being seen for his first interview by a woman therapist. Frank was suffering from a depression, having been jilted by his girlfriend. In describing his girlfriend, Frank referred to her as "cold" and "critical." Later in the interview he referred to his mother as "dominating" and "unappreciative." Discussing his work place, he mentioned that his boss, a woman, had him "by the balls."

Although Frank's interviewer clearly saw the theme running through all of Frank's relationships with women, she did not realize that Frank was experiencing her the same way. Frank did not return for a second appointment.

What is important to keep in mind during the first and subsequent interviews as well is that whom the patient talks about is usually a reference in one way or another to the therapist (Brenner 1976, Freud 1904). If the therapist does not recognize this and does not show his understanding of this fact to the patient, then termination of the contact is eminently possible. Yet if the therapist relates openly and directly to transferential material, particularly when it suggests resistance and negative feelings, it can make it more probable for the patient to return for more therapeutic contact.

Frank, in the above case illustration, went to see another female therapist a few weeks later. Not only did he again describe his girlfriend, mother, and boss in similar terms, but he labeled the previous therapist he had seen as "a cold potato." This time the therapist, after feeling that she too was about to be rejected any moment, said to Frank, "Frank, I see that you have been given a hard time by lots of women. I wonder if you are feeling any of this right now with me?" Frank heaved a sigh of relief and said, "I'm really glad you asked me that! I was wondering when you were going to say something sadistic. I guess I'm always ready for that from a woman. You know, when you asked me that question, I started to feel understood and began to like you." Frank did stay in treatment with the second therapist.

Since potential patients are frequently eager to find love, they often come to the first interview hoping to find a loving person. This can take the form of flattering the therapist and saying all kinds of laudatory things about him. It is important to remember that as empathetic and competent as the therapist may be, these are also *transference reactions*, designed to get a response from the practitioner. If the practitioner is made uncomfortable by the flattery and tries to deflect it, or takes it too seriously and becomes too grateful for it, the patient will feel misunderstood and may terminate.

> Gloria, a married woman in her thirties, sought help because she was feeling guilty about being involved in an extramarital affair. After discussing her marriage for while, she turned to the male therapist and said, "You're a very patient and empathetic man." The therapist, uncomfortable with the praise, changed the subject. When Gloria later in the interview said, "You're the type of man I'd like to have an affair with," the therapist blushed and said, "Thank you very much, but this is a professional relationship." Gloria ended the session before the time was up, feeling very rejected.
>
> In her next contact with a therapist, also a male, Gloria tried again to be seductive and ingratiating. In this contact, the therapist responded to her transference reactions and commented, "I get the feeling you have felt insufficiently loved. I also get the impression that this is something you'd like my help with." Gloria very much appreciated the therapist's attentiveness and remained in treatment.

COUNTERTRANSFERENCE REACTIONS
DURING THE FIRST INTERVIEW

Countertransference, "all of the therapist's reactions to the patient, which may help or hinder treatment" (Slakter 1987, p. 3), like transference, is everpresent. It must be studied constantly by all practitioners (Brenner 1985). One of the difficulties in studying countertransference reactions is that their meaning usually comes to us in hindsight (Renik 1993). Just as the patient is not consciously aware of distorting the therapist when she does so, the same applies to the practitioner. Usually he's not aware of his countertransference reactions until after the session, and sometimes many sessions later.

A fairly common countertransference reaction is to want to rescue the patient (Maroda 1994, Searles 1979). The reason this is a frequent reaction among therapists is that virtually all of them have suffered a great deal during their own lives (Sussman 1992) and would have loved someone to rescue them. By trying to rescue the patient, the therapist feels in many ways that he is being rescued (A. Freud 1946).

Howard, a 19-year-old college student, was being seen for his first interview at a student mental health center. He was quite depressed, felt rejected by everybody on the college campus, and at times thought of committing suicide. As his female therapist listened to his plight, she felt extremely sorry for him and during the course of the session had wishes to "mother" him. Fortunately, she could monitor these wishes because when Howard asked her to talk to some of his professors and "intercede," she could study his request rather than gratify it.

Because Howard's request was frustrated, he could discharge a little anger. Feeling less tense, he felt helped by his interviewer and continued to come to see her.

During the first interview, countertransference can take many forms. When one feels unsure of himself and worried about impressing the prospective patient, he can make many interpretations and try to show how smart he is. When the therapist feels like being a rescuer, intervening in the environment is often a way of expressing the rescue fantasy. Countertransference, like transference, must always be studied in order not to act out one's subjective wishes and anxieties.

ANSWERING QUESTIONS IN THE FIRST INTERVIEW

In the last chapter we discussed the issue of answering the patient's questions. While the same principles hold, there are certain questions that are frequently asked during the course of the first interview that need special attention.

One question that prospective patients often ask near the end of the first interview is, "What do you think is the matter with me?" If the patient is sophisticated and acculturated, she may ask, "What is your diagnosis and prognosis?" When the patient is involved in an interpersonal conflict with a spouse, parent, child, or significant other, she may ask, "How much of this problem is mine? Do you think it's all my fault?"

Although some clinicians contend that the patient has a right to hear her diagnosis and prognosis, I believe questions about the therapist's dynamic assessment reflect the patient's anxiety about how disturbed she is. Therefore, instead of answering these questions, the reasons they are being asked should be investigated.

> Isabelle, a married woman in her early forties, was being seen for her first interview by a male therapist. After Isabelle spent considerable time describing many of her marital conflicts, in which she and her husband alternated between yelling and screaming and then not talking to each other, Isabelle asked the therapist, "What do you think is going on between my husband and me?" The therapist responded by saying, "I think you two are involved in a power struggle."
>
> Although the therapist's impression seemed to be correct, Isabelle did not like his comment and stated, "You think I'm just as crazy as he is?" When the therapist didn't respond to this, Isabelle's fury grew intense and she ended the interview by pointing out that she felt very misunderstood by the therapist and was not coming back.

As we have stressed, despite the fact that patients are suffering, they have a strong desire to maintain the status quo and almost always have much resistance to learning about themselves. Consequently, it is more helpful for patients to discover maladaptive behavior by themselves, rather than to have it pointed out to them, particularly in the early interviews.

When Isabelle saw another practitioner a few weeks later, she told the female therapist similar vignettes about her dysfunctional interactions with her husband. Also similar to her previous experience with the male therapist, at the end of the interview she asked, "What do you think is going on with me and my husband?" This therapist said, "I know you'd like me to answer your question but it might be helpful for us to see what you are feeling right now when you ask me this question." After a pause Isabelle said, "I'm worried you'll think everything is my fault and then think very little of me." The therapist then responded, "I think you're ready to have me give you a hard time and hit you hard." Isabelle then said, "I'm always ready to be in a fight. It happens a lot to me. I think I have to talk about this some more with you." Isabelle did return for more therapy and sustained her contact for over a year.

One question that is also asked frequently during the course of the first interview is, "What is your fee?" I do believe that this question has to be answered!

As most experienced clinicians know, when the therapist says, "My usual fee is $___ a session," not all prospective patients respond by saying "That's fine. I'm ready to pay that fee." Many prospective patients try to negotiate with the therapist about lowering the fee and a bargaining session then ensues.

I believe that bargaining sessions do not help create the appropriate atmosphere for the first interview (or for any other interview). Yet the reason I think they are so plentiful is because clinicians are often reluctant to explore their prospective patients' financial situation. Many years ago therapists and patients avoided discussing sex. Since the sexual revolution, the fear of talking about sex has been replaced by a resistance to discussing money.

When a prospective patient voices reluctance to pay my usual fee, I ask, "Perhaps we should take a look at your finances?" This returns the interview into an investigative one and patient and therapist can then begin to understand how much basis there is in reality for the patient's resistance to paying the therapist's usual fee.

Although prospective patients sometimes exhibit shame and embarrassment when they are asked about their finances (responding as if they were asked to disrobe and show something private), most patients welcome a frank discussion of money, and therapist and patient can then make a more informed decision about the fee based on a sound exploration of the patient's real and fantasied financial assets.

Jack, in his early thirties, sought treatment because he was having difficulty getting along with his superiors in the accounting firm in which he was employed. In his first interview with a male therapist, he was able to talk openly and spontaneously about his problems and related positively to the therapist. However, near the end of the interview when Jack asked the therapist what he would be charged for therapy and he was told the fee, which was not excessive, Jack said, "I could never afford that!"

When the therapist empathized with Jack's inability to afford the requested fee and then asked Jack what he thought he could afford, Jack suggested that he be charged one-half of the amount the therapist had requested. The therapist then suggested, "Let's take a look at your income and expenses and see what we can work out together." Jack went into a long silence and then said, "I don't know why I'm so tight. I make over $100,000 a year." Subsequently he went into a prolonged discussion on why he was always "counting pennies" and concluded that money was an issue that he needed to discuss further with the therapist.

With the possible exception of answering the prospective patient's question about the fee, I believe most questions asked during the first interview should be explored rather than answered. Many of the questions asked in the first interview will be similar to those that some prospective patients asked during the initial phone conversation. Questions about the therapist's credentials, his theoretical orientation, preferred treatment modality, religion, or sexual orientation will appear again—and again. A most expedient method of responding to most queries is to investigate what the patient is feeling when she asks them.

CANCELING THE FIRST INTERVIEW

Until now we have assumed that after a positive phone conversation, the prospective patient will keep the appointment for her first interview. However, this is not always the case. A certain percentage of patients become frightened of a face-to-face interview and do not show up. Some call to cancel, and some do not.

All too often therapists try to convince a reluctant applicant to come in for an interview. On doing this, they overlook the fact that this posture exacerbates the individual's mistrust and compounds her resistance. Resistive individuals need to feel they have a right to resist treatment. When the practitioner empathically notes that beginning treatment might be something that the person would prefer to avoid right now, this compassionate attitude often frees the reluctant applicant to view psychotherapy more favorably.

Most prospective patients respond positively when a clinician is not critical of patients who don't show up for the initial interview. The individual's manifest statement, even though a defensive one, should be respected and it should be borne in mind that sometimes accidents do occur, and traffic snarls do take place. What is crucial for the prospective patient who resists coming to the first interview is a clinician who is accepting and not critical, understanding and nonjudgmental. Consequently, when a prospective patient cancels the first appointment, she should be told that it was regrettable that an interview couldn't take place, but perhaps another can be scheduled soon.

Those clients who call the therapist after they cancel the first appointment are usually less resistive than those who do not, and often do come for another interview. However, those who do not call are usually very frightened people who need much patience and care before they can feel free to come in for a face-to-face session. A phone call that is not pressuring but understanding of how difficult it is to begin treatment may help them consider having an interview. What is most helpful to these individuals is a therapist's attitude that conveys the message that they can take plenty of time before coming in for a first interview.

RELUCTANCE TO GIVE INFORMATION

Particularly during the initial interviews therapists want to get some information about the prospective patient's symptoms, ego functions, superego mandates, interpersonal problems, history, and so forth. Although most individuals are willing to answer the therapist's questions about their past and present circumstances, many are reluctant to discuss certain facets of their lives. Almost all patients have some secret or secrets they do not want to divulge, particularly in their early interviews. I had a patient whom I saw four times a week who did not tell me his name for a year (Strean 1991). I've had at least three patients who were in treatment over two years before they could share and analyze a dream (Strean 1998) and I've had many patients who withheld fantasies, memories, and other facets of their lives for very long periods of time.

As we have suggested, entering psychotherapy is often experienced as being relegated to an ignoble, submissive position in which one has lost control and power; one way of restoring control and power is by withholding information from the clinician (Noble and Hamilton 1983).

Since a refusal to give information to the clinician is an obvious form of resistance, its occurrence affords the therapist an excellent opportunity to demonstrate early in therapy how the phenomenon of resistance is addressed. If the therapist responds sensitively, confidently, and empathically to the patient's reluctance to give information, this attitude will help the patient feel less self-conscious and anxious. On the other hand, if the patient feels pressured to reveal information, she will become progressively more uncomfortable and will probably leave treatment.

> A teenager of 15, Kermit was referred to a mental health clinic by the courts because he had been convicted of stealing. In his intake interview with the social worker, he refused to discuss the details of his stealing. When the social worker told Kermit that he couldn't be helped with his problems if he didn't tell her what had happened, he became more provocative and said, "I'll go to jail then!"
>
> In a later interview with a different professional, when Kermit was again reluctant to talk about the details of his stealing, the therapist said, "If it's too tough to talk about, don't tell me now. But I would like to understand better what you'd feel if you did tell me." Kermit responded by saying, "I don't like to be put down by anybody. You're the big shot here and I resent it." The therapist empathized with Kermit's plight and said, "I guess the more you tell me, the stronger I get and the less you tell me the stronger you get." Kermit felt understood and the treatment continued.

What is important for both prospective patient and therapist to realize is that when a patient has difficulty revealing material, she feels in danger, and it is the dangerous situation that needs to be understood by both of them.

GROUND RULES AND
THE FIRST INTERVIEW

All therapists, regardless of their theoretical predilections and preferred therapeutic modalities, have ground rules for their practices (Langs 1973). Policies about absences, payments, discussing the therapy with others, and other issues are necessary to provide stability, continuity, and value to the treatment. While ground rules differ from therapist to therapist and their defiance by either therapist or patient needs to be controlled and mastered, we are concerned here with the issues of ground rules as they pertain to the first interview.

If a patient asks me my policies about missed sessions, vacations, or some other ground rule during the first session, first I will try to find out what's on the patient's mind that prompts her to ask. Often I don't have to announce the ground rule because the patient's feelings, fantasies, and anxieties that prompted the question move to the forefront. But, for example, if the patient's work requires her to be out of town a lot, or she can only take vacations at specified times, we obviously need to work out a plan that satisfies each of us. My usual ground rule for absences is that I will try to make up the absence if I know about it with sufficient notice, but if I can't change her appointment or fill her time I will charge the patient for it.

What I like to avoid in the first interview is prematurely announcing ground rules. If the issue does not come up, why raise an obstacle? Otherwise I can appear like a disciplinarian and most patients have quite a bit of intolerance toward people in authority. By telling prospective patients rules they have to follow before a relationship is formed, I can stir up negative feelings in them and interfere with the formation of a working alliance. Rather, I prefer to wait for the first cancellation or some other disruption of the therapy, study the psychological and reality issues, then explain that I will not charge for this absence, but then explain what my policy is.

> Larry, an attorney, had to be out of town during his sixth month of treatment as part of his work. When he returned, his therapist said, "I won't charge you for the missed session because you don't know my policy about fees. In the future, if we can make up the absence or I can fill the hour, I won't charge you. Otherwise, I'll have to charge." Larry responded, "That's reasonable," and adapted to the ground rule quite easily.

If the therapist appears reasonable and caring, listens most of the time, and asks pertinent questions at strategic moments, most first interviews go well. The therapist should try to monitor his wishes to give advice, make interpretations, intervene in the patient's environment, and announce ground rules. If the therapist is successful in emerging as an empathetic listener, the patient is readied to form a positive therapeutic alliance.

CHAPTER THREE

Understanding the Honeymoon Phase of Treatment and Becoming a Competent Honeymooner

The main task for the therapist in the early phase of treatment is to help the patient want to stay in treatment; everything else is of secondary importance. The therapist's major focus during this time, therefore, is to determine what facilitates and what impedes the formation of a positive relationship between the patient and the therapist (Fine 1982).

As we have stated, the best way to ensure that the patient will stay in treatment is to listen carefully to her. Inexperienced and insufficiently trained therapists have considerable difficulty in genuinely believing this important axiom of practice, and many of those clinicians who accept the validity of this tenet do not find it easy to practice! Listening to the patient's material without interrupting her frequently assumes that the therapist feels sufficiently competent so that he doesn't have to show how clever he is by producing brilliant comments, probing questions, and creative advice. It also suggests that the therapist can listen to material without being made to feel too anxious by it. Finally, a belief in the importance of listening to the patient implies a faith in the patient's capacity to feel more valued as a person when she is quietly accepted by an attentive and empathetic listener.

When the patient does most of the talking and the therapist does most of the listening, a working alliance is usually formed (Greenson 1967). In a working alliance, the healthy part of the patient's ego joins with the healthy part of the therapist's ego to uncover and resolve the maladaptive and neurotic parts of the patient. If treatment is to be successful, the working alliance must be maintained throughout the treatment process. The negative transference and negative countertransference, as well as other resistances and counterresistances, tend to destroy the working alliance; consequently, the practitioner must be particularly vigilant to those behaviors of the patient and himself that oppose the treatment and each other. This is particularly true during the beginning phase of therapy.

If the therapist listens attentively and encourages the patient to talk freely, the patient begins to develop warm and loving feelings toward the therapist. Although there are a few exceptions to this therapeutic postulate, most patients find that an empathetic listener induces in them the feeling that they are similar to a loved son or daughter who has a parent who loves them unconditionally. When the patient talks and is not censured, not criticized, not corrected or advised, she begins to feel that the therapist is the equivalent of a benign superego. Accepted by a benign superego, the patient begins to accept herself more and more.

Another benefit that accrues when the patient primarily talks and the therapist spends most of his time listening is patient catharsis. This involves the patient's unburdening herself of guilty thoughts and feelings, shameful self-images, forbidden actions, and embarrassing moments. The catharsis is, of course, ensured when the therapist attentively listens without interruption. When the patient feels unburdened, her self-esteem rises as she finds herself in a new and enabling relationship.

As the benefits of talking to a warm listener mount, the patient usually enters into a "honeymoon." Feeling loved and valued, she begins to love. Experiencing an "unconditional positive regard" (Rogers 1951) emanating from the therapist, the patient begins to regard the therapist very positively and, feeling that the therapist offers hope, the patient with the therapist's support looks forward to a pleasant future with the therapist at her side.

Although honeymoons do not endure forever, they do provide the partners with feelings of hope and security because the partners realize that they have demonstrated the capacity of loving each other and working together productively. Therefore, it is incumbent on the practitioner to help the patient move toward a honeymoon and reap some of its therapeutic benefit.

In this chapter, our aim will be to study those issues that interfere with the development and continuation of a honeymoon. We shall concern ourselves with those resistances that both partners bring but, as is true throughout this text, we will place a heavier emphasis on the therapist's role in facilitating a honeymoon.

TO LOVE OR NOT TO LOVE: THAT IS THE QUESTION

Most dynamically oriented therapists take the position that what primarily motivates men and women to enter psychotherapy are dissatisfactions with their ability to love and be loved (Fine 1985, Kernberg 1995). Furthermore, most practitioners have as their primary objective to help the patient reduce her hatred and increase her capacity to love (Fine 1982). In order to become more loving, the patient has to be able to love the therapist with more freedom as the treatment proceeds, and to be able concomitantly to accept his love.

Why do people have difficulty in loving? Countless psychoanalytic and psychotherapy books and articles have been written on the subject (for example, Bergmann 1987, Gabbard 1996). Furthermore, from time immemorial, poets, novelists, and others have spent much thought and energy as they have discussed what impedes and facilitates love. But, first, what is love? As an old song goes, "Love is a dream. Hard to explain just how you feel. Deep in your heart, joy seems to dwell. . . ."

Love, then, is a product in part of fantasies. As in a dream, we experience the loved one as having qualities that bring us joy. And our joy induces joy in the partner. Love, to be sustained, must be mutual.

The writer who explained more clearly and more comprehensively than any other researcher why we can't love is Sigmund Freud. Freud (1905) demonstrated quite convincingly that to understand the vicissitudes of love, we have to sensitize ourselves to the child that exists in every adult. As we examine our patient's psychosexual development, we observe what interferes with her capacity to love. For example, if the patient as an infant did not receive consistent tender love and care she will not be able to trust another human being sufficiently and will become quite paranoid

(Erikson 1950). Or as a child the patient may have been used by a parent to compensate for his or her own dissatisfactions with marriage and other aspects of life, smothering the youngster. This then induces in the child a wish to flee from relationships because they appear too engulfing. Many parents provide an atmosphere that creates shame and doubt (Erikson 1950) in their children as they squelch the spontaneous expression of instinctual impulses. Finally, many family situations are such that mother and father exploit their children as they fight it out with each other and use their children as allies. This kind of setting creates problems in sexual identity, interpersonal relations, and self-esteem when the child becomes an adult.

Most of the problems that the child experiences in growing up emerge when she becomes an adult in the psychotherapeutic relationship with the therapist. As the therapist benignly listens with empathy and without censure, many patients fear their growing dependency feelings and are impelled to become more autonomous very quickly. As the therapist does not judge or take sides, many patients become troubled by sexual and aggressive impulses toward him and become very inhibited and secretive in the treatment situation. As the therapist shows warmth and understanding, the patient may feel guilt as she experiences oedipal and incestuous fantasies toward him.

Inasmuch as therapists are "more human than otherwise" (Sullivan 1953) they, too, are not exempt from having fears and anxieties about intimacy that interfere with the development of a honeymoon. It should be noted that sometimes the patient is more capable of being a honeymooner than the therapist (Sussman 1992), who may become uncomfortable when the patient's dependency wishes and other yearnings for intimacy appear.

During the beginning stages of therapy, the patient's warm, positive, and loving feelings should be accepted and not questioned. What needs attention during the early months of treatment are the subtle and not-so-subtle signs of negative transference because of the patient's anxiety about loving and being loved. Let us look more carefully at some specific resistances that emerge during the early phases of treatment.

FEAR OF DEPENDENCY

One of the most frequent resistances noted during the early phases of treatment is the patient's fear of depending on the therapist. Many patients, because of their forbidden wish to regress and become a small toddler again with a loving parent completely taking care of them, have to fight the idea of being in therapy. Particularly men who have to be macho often cope with the idea of being in the dependent patient role by criticizing the therapist and/or trying to get him into an argument about the pros and cons of being in therapy.

One of the best ways to lose a patient is to get into an argument with her and try to convince her that she needs therapy and should depend on the therapist. Many therapists, particularly those who work in clinics and agencies, take a judgmental position on "poorly motivated" patients and criticize them for opposing treatment. When they do this they fail to recognize that when patients resist something, they feel they are in danger. Unless the therapist relates to the danger, the patient will leave treatment.

Annabelle, in her early thirties, was seen in a mental health center because her 8-year-old daughter had a severe school phobia. When Annabelle was told in the first interview by her therapist, Mr. B., that they would meet weekly, Annabelle aggressively asked, "Do we have to meet every single week?" Mr. B. responded authoritatively and directly with a resounding, "Yes, that's the policy of our treatment center!" To this, Annabelle queried, "Could you explain your policy to me?" Mr. B. then gave a clear and comprehensive explanation of how it was important for the child's treatment for the parent to be helped "to sustain the child's gains" and "to determine how the parent can better facilitate the child's development."

Annabelle continued to ask many more questions and Mr. B. continued to give many more answers. After the session, Annabelle asked for an appointment with the chief social worker, Ms. C., in order to complain about Mr. B.

Ms. C. told Annabelle that possibly there was something wrong with the center's policy and maybe it needed to be corrected. She encouraged Annabelle to discuss all of her doubts and criticisms about the policy and welcomed her expressions of anger. Annabelle agreed to come in regularly to see Ms. C. if she would not be regarded as a patient and "the meetings" would be viewed as "educational" for Ms. C.

Inasmuch as Ms. C. did not argue with Annabelle but could accept her wrath and criticisms, "non-patient"

Annabelle continued to see Ms. C. Eventually, she found herself feeling "very fond" of Ms. C. and in her fourth month of the contact, began to discuss some of her own problems.

WISHES FOR DEPENDENCY GRATIFICATION

As was suggested earlier, in most cases in the treatment situation, with its emphasis on being helped, the "child" in the adult patient emerges rather early. Sometimes, as in the case of Annabelle, the patient defends against her childish dependency feelings. This requires the therapist to be respectful of the patient's resistance and not try to talk her into becoming a patient, as Mr. B., Annabelle's first therapist, attempted to do. While many patients fight their dependency wishes, others do the opposite and try to "milk" the therapist as much as possible. They insist on trying to get the therapist to give them advice on how to conduct their lives, join with them against their enemies, tell them how lovable they are, and speak to them on the phone between sessions.

If the therapist gets manipulated into seeing himself as an always available breast, he will soon discover that the patient will become insatiable and he will become exhausted. On the other hand, if the patient's dependency wishes are too quickly frustrated or subtly condemned, the patient will leave treatment in a rage.

David, a married man in his mid-fifties, was in treatment with Ms. E., a private practitioner. David sought therapy because his wife was "always criticizing and demeaning" him and this made him alternately "depressed and very angry."

In the treatment situation, David very much appreciated Ms. E.'s "compassionate and caring" attitude. Within a few sessions his depression "vanished" and he no longer found himself getting angry either. David very much liked Ms. E.'s "warm and quiet demeanor" and he found it "wonderful just to talk."

By the second month of therapy David was telling Ms.E. that she was both "the mother and the wife" that he always wanted. He began to ask Ms. E. for advice about how to handle his wife and Ms. E. soon found herself accommodating her patient. The advice was "so helpful" that David began to seek it in between his weekly sessions by calling Ms. E. frequently. The phone calls mounted as did the requests for advice. Eventually Ms. E. became exasperated and began to be somewhat curt and withholding in her responses to David. This aroused David's anger and soon he became as depressed as he had appeared when he began treatment. He threatened to leave treatment and even thought of suicide.

Feeling desperate, Ms. E. sought consultation from a senior colleague. As she examined her countertransference reactions, she realized that she had felt very flattered by David's deep gratitude and genuine appreciation of her. Consequently, she was not able to explore with David what he was feeling when he asked for advice or sought her out in between sessions. Ms. E. wanted to maintain David's love and was afraid of his aggression. When Ms. E. could confront her own narcissism, she was able to become more of a therapist to David and less of a feeding mother and nurturing wife.

By the fifth month of treatment Ms. E. assumed a more helpful therapeutic stance with David. First, she shared with him that she had not been helpful to him by giving him constant advice in and out of sessions because it made him lose confidence in himself. Second, she told David that she thought it would be a good idea to see what David was feeling and thinking when he wanted advice or needed to call Ms. E. on the phone. Although David was quite petulant at first, he was able to voice his anger at Ms. E. for withholding "valuable nutrition." He began to compare her with his mother and wife who "could not nurture" him.

As David could express some of his dissatisfactions with Ms. E., his marital relationship improved. Eventually he could confront how very ambivalent he had felt toward his own mother. To ward off the hatred he felt toward his mother and to escape the doubts he had about her loving him, David needed constant reassurance. The more he faced this issue, the more mature he could become in all of his relationships, including his therapeutic relationship with Ms. E.

In the early stages of therapy, it is extremely important for the therapist to be sensitive to the patient's resistances against depending on the therapist as well as to what Freud (1939) called *id resistances*—attempts by the patient to have the therapist gratify childish dependency wishes. When the therapist relates to the patient's difficulties with dependency, the patient feels more comfortable about depending on him.

SEXUAL ISSUES

When the patient feels loved and cared for by the therapist, inevitably sexual fantasies are aroused in her. The therapeutic situation, where the patient is given carte blanche to say everything that comes to mind with an empathetic person listening, is a most inviting atmosphere for the arousal of sexual fantasies. Although the sexual revolution has made it more permissible for patients and therapists to discuss sexual feelings toward each other, it is still an anxiety-provoking situation for many.

One of the reasons that a discussion of sexual issues is difficult for so many individuals is that sexual feelings and fantasies (like dependency wishes) have many childish components. The reason that adults are embarrassed to discuss sexual fantasies is that they feel like children getting undressed and/or watching somebody else doing the same. Therefore, sexual feelings, which are often forbidden for children to experience, are often felt to be a forbidden topic in therapy. Many therapists and many patients do not permit themselves to entertain sexual fantasies toward each other. Like guilt-ridden children, sex can be a taboo subject for them.

Yet a good honeymoon is one where sex is a mutually enjoyable experience. Therefore, the honeymoon phase of treatment should contain some discussion of sex. However, as we have implied, because it arouses anxiety, patients and therapists have different ways to inhibit discussion of the subject.

Just as children who are aroused sexually can attack those to whom they are attracted (Offit 1995), many patients and therapists can become critical or hostile toward each other to ward off feeling their sexual impulses. And just as many individuals who fear their sexual fantasies flee from the place or person who arouses them, many patients who flee treatment are running away from sexual excitement. Particularly when therapist and patient are the same gender, this can be a very anxiety-ridden issue.

> Florence, a 17-year-old high school senior, was in therapy with Dr. G., a female psychologist working in a mental health center. Florence was being seen because she was in constant arguments with her mother, whom she experienced as very controlling.
>
> During the first few weeks of therapy, Florence spoke at length of her conflicts with her mother, and released a lot of anger toward her. After she had several catharses, she began to become very interested in Dr. G.'s clothes, her jewelry, and often complimented Dr. G. on her good taste. Dr. G. did not place any particular significance on Florence's preoccupation with her clothes and was very surprised when Florence, during the second month of treatment, wanted to quit therapy.
>
> As Dr. G. reviewed her treatment of Florence in supervision, she became aware of the fact that her patient's interest in Dr. G.'s clothes and jewelry was really a displacement of her interest in Dr. G.'s body. By Dr. G. not responding to Florence's interest, Florence felt like a rejected lover. Moreover, Dr. G. was able to realize that she had been defending against her own sexual attraction to Florence.

In later sessions, when Dr. G. told Florence that she hadn't paid sufficient attention to Florence's interest in clothes, Florence showed visible appreciation. Therapist and patient could then discuss how Florence's mother was unavailable to talk about a "girl's interests." This eventually led to a discussion about Florence's preferences in clothes and perfumes. Feeling understood, Florence could then share her curiosity with Dr. G. about sexual matters such as birth control, menstruation, and other sexual subjects. This helped Florence stay in treatment.

Not sufficiently recognized as a manifestation of the honeymoon transference is the patient's increased sexual activity during the beginning phase of therapy. Many patients, rather than express their sexual fantasies (homosexual or heterosexual) directly toward the therapist, become involved in one or more sexual affairs. Two common errors that clinicians make when confronted by a patient's increased sexual activity are: (1) to become unduly alarmed and try to get the patient to curb her sexual activity; or (2) vicariously to enjoy the patient's activity, encourage fuller participation in sex by the patient, but without an understanding of what the patient is experiencing internally.

It is never helpful to a patient, particularly during the beginning phase of treatment, to oppose her behavior. Feeling pressured to repress her wishes, the patient either complies and suffers or retaliates and quits treatment. To encourage a patient to behave in a certain way, such as to have sexual liaisons, is initially titillating to both parties, but eventually the patient feels used and the therapist feels frustrated. The best stance when a patient embarks on an affair, which is almost always a displacement of the current transference towards the therapist, is to help the patient eventually discover that she is acting out the transference and to help her see why she is doing so.

> When Hal, a married man in his early forties, embarked on an extramarital affair during his third month of treatment, his male therapist, Dr. I., showed interest but delayed commenting on it. Eventually Hal told Dr. I. that he thought the latter disapproved of his having an extramarital affair. When this perception was explored, Hal said that he wanted the therapist's permission to have an extramarital affair because the romance started when he began therapy. On Dr. I.'s asking Hal what he thought had been going on in their work that got Hal interested in an affair, Hal spoke about the "good feeling" he was having with Dr. I. at his side. Eventually Hal had several homosexual dreams that involved sex between him and the therapist. The homosexuality was an expression of Hal's deep yearning to be close to his father. Feeling frightened of these feelings toward his father substitute, Dr. I., Hal had an affair with a woman who unconsciously stood for the woman in himself who wanted contact with his father.

When the patient's sexual wishes are neither praised nor condemned, neither encouraged nor discouraged, she has a good opportunity to examine her feelings and see just what they are all about. This requires the therapist to view his own sexuality and his patient's as facts of life. Anna Freud's (1946) "equidistant" approach is particularly pertinent to the treatment of sexual issues. By "equidistant" Anna Freud meant that the therapist neither champions nor deplores the patient's id wishes, superego commands, or ego defenses. Rather, he shows the patient how the various parts of her psyche are interacting, such as was done in the treatment of Hal in the above case illustration.

AGGRESSIVE ISSUES

Most people who seek psychotherapy have difficulty with their aggression. Many patients are so afraid they will inflict either psychological or physical harm on others if they release their aggression that they turn their aggression inward, becoming very self-effacing and masochistic. Others show a pattern of repressing and suppressing aggression for long periods of time and then have a violent outburst that gets them into trouble with others and with themselves.

During the early stages of treatment when the patient is encouraged to talk about anything that is on her mind, sooner or later (and usually sooner) she finds herself talking about angry feelings toward family members and others. Sometimes these are hostile reactions that are still simmering from the past, and at other times they are hostile thoughts and fantasies toward individuals in their current reality. As the therapist does not censure expressions of anger, some patients accept this as permission to ventilate more and more anger (catharses) without guilt. This enables their self-esteem to rise and they can feel more competent and assertive in their interpersonal relationships.

One of the main reasons patients have difficulty in normally asserting themselves is because as they make a request, disagree with someone, or say "no," they are worried that hostile fantasies will erupt and be discharged. Many patients need to be helped to see that they tend to equate fantasies with actions. Then they can't like themselves very much. This kind of confusion can emerge during the early phase of treatment between patient and therapist.

> Jane, in her early thirties, was in her second month of treatment in a family agency. She was being seen primarily because she felt very depressed about her unsatisfactory marriage.
>
> When her social worker, Ms. K., realized that Jane was depressed in her marriage because she had repressed and suppressed much of her hostility toward her husband, she tried to encourage Jane to express some of it in the sessions. Jane denied having any hostility toward her husband and became even more depressed than she had been when she entered treatment.
>
> After Ms. K. discussed the case with a senior colleague, she realized that Jane was angry at her for confronting Jane with hostility toward her husband—something that was too dangerous for Jane to deal with. When Ms. K. told Jane that she thought she had upset her by talking with her about her anger toward her husband, Jane denied it. This then led to a discussion between therapist and patient about how frightening it was to talk about angry feelings in general—

something that was always prohibited in Jane's family of origin.

When Ms. K. tried less to get Jane to ventilate her anger but tried more to help her discuss her fears of it, Jane became much more comfortable in the treatment encounter. After several sessions of examining her fears of hostility and seeing how she erroneously viewed a hostile thought as a hostile deed, Jane was eventually able to be more assertive with Ms. K. and with her husband, and not feel so guilty about doing so.

Just as therapists can vicariously derive pleasure from their patients' sexual activity and subtly encourage it, they can do the same thing with their patients' hostile outbursts toward parents, employers, spouses, colleagues, and friends. What can happen during the beginning phase of treatment is that the patient and therapist form an alliance wherein they jointly demean an adversary of the patient's as they support each other. This can lead to a premature ending of treatment because most patients would rather divorce a therapist that they know for a couple of months than abandon a spouse or employer toward whom they are ambivalent but to whom they have been attached for several years.

Larry was a single man in his early forties who was seeing Dr. M., a male therapist in private practice. Larry sought treatment because he wanted to separate from his parents, with whom he had been living all of his life.

During the first three months of treatment, Larry complained a great deal about his parents' extreme dependency on him, their unwillingness to let him have a life of his own, and their total inability to permit him to have angry feelings toward them.

In response to Larry's comments about his relationship with his parents, Dr. M. encouraged Larry to discuss his angry feelings toward them. Initially, Larry derived a lot of gratification from the therapist's support, but by the fifth month of treatment, Larry began to come late for sessions, held back his payment of fees, and threatened to quit treatment.

What Dr. M. was able to discover when he realized that Larry did not feel helped, was that he was not relating to his patient's ambivalence toward his parents. Yes, Larry felt hostility toward his parents, but he also loved them. Therefore, when Dr. M. encouraged the expression of hostility toward Larry's parents, Larry felt very guilty and wanted to get away from Dr. M.

Inasmuch as Dr. M. could help Larry see why his hostility toward his parents bothered him so much—it was as if Larry were "knocking off" his parents whom he valued—the therapy could progress.

In order to help patients deal with their aggressive drives during the beginning phase of treatment, it is important for the therapist to realize that the expression of aggression is only part of a process, not an end in itself. Patients need to see that it is frightening to hate someone they also love. Furthermore, one of the tasks of therapy that can only be briefly introduced in the beginning phase of treatment is that anger that is held onto reflects unresolved problems with dependency, narcissism, sexuality, and other issues that will eventually have to be addressed, but later into the treatment. If the therapist embarks on this too soon, the patient will fight it.

THE PREMATURE SEARCH
FOR DYNAMIC MATERIAL

Particularly during the beginning of treatment, when the individual feels inhibited and defensive, there is a tendency on the part of many patients to talk obsessively about mundane subjects and avoid facing their problems and their feelings. I remember listening twice a week for several months to a man who discussed every item of every meal he ate, and nothing else. I recall a woman who for several months several times a week described the minutiae of her everyday life such as brushing her teeth, taking a shower, going to the toilet, eating breakfast. And I shall never forget working in a child guidance clinic with a mother who spent her sessions describing every one of her son's bowel movements!

Because I was very bored and also felt I wasn't earning my fee, I tried to help these patients express the feelings, fantasies, and memories that were underneath their obsessions. My patients resisted almost all of my attempts and in response to my showing insufficient respect for their defenses, they became more defensive and threatened to leave treatment.

One of the best ways to facilitate a working alliance is to begin where the patient is. If the patient continually wants to talk about meals, bowel movements, and such, the therapist must remind himself that any other focus would threaten the patient too much. It is only by respecting the patient's resistances that we can expect positive results. It is always good to remind ourselves that patients resist to avoid danger.

Jack was a senior citizen, in his early seventies. He had just retired from a university position, where he had been very successful as a chemistry professor. His purpose in seeking treatment was "to try to cope better," since his retirement from teaching induced in him acute boredom and depression.

When Jack began therapy with Ms. K., a therapist in private practice, he did not discuss his boredom at all, nor did he mention his depression. What he did do was talk about his activities as an officer in the army during World War II. He regaled Ms. K. with stories exhibiting his leadership skills and ability to win friends and influence people.

Ms. K. realized quite early in her contact with Jack that to compensate for his depressed feelings and current low self-esteem, Jack had to exhibit his vitality and military prowess. As Jack was not interrupted with questions or interpretations, he began to feel warmly toward Ms. K. As Jack felt valued, his self-esteem improved and his depression diminished. After feeling supported and accepted, Jack could turn to a discussion of his problems.

It is never a waste of time for a therapist to respect a patient's resistances—particularly during the early phases of treatment. When the patient feels unthreatened and not questioned, she is much more likely to form a therapeutic alliance and move into a positive transference.

AVOIDING THE TRANSFERENCE

I know of no concept that assists the mental health practitioner more than the notion of transference. When Freud (1912) introduced the concept of transference, he viewed it as those reactions of the patient, conscious and unconscious, to the therapist that emanate from the patient's past. Recognizing that this phenomenon is always at work and is not unique to psychotherapy, but is a universal phenomenon occurring in all human relationships, helps the clinician understand better why at different times he is loved, hated, and treated ambivalently or indifferently.

What modern therapists now recognize is that there is not a one-to-one correspondence between how the patient perceived a figure in the past and how she experiences the therapist in the present. For example, the therapist may be experienced as the embodiment of all that the patient wishes a perfect parent to be, or the therapist may be experienced as the devalued self-image of the patient and thus scapegoated. In effect, many times the therapist is perceived through the lens of the patient's fantasies.

In the therapeutic situation, particularly in the early stages of it, the transference reactions are often expressed subtly and indirectly. The patient may be talking of an ambivalently experienced teacher but is unconsciously referring to the therapist. Or the patient may refer to a friend or relative who is in psychotherapy and describe her relationship to her therapist, but she really is giving the current therapist all kinds of prescriptions and proscriptions. Very often the patient's references to those charged with helping others are descriptions of the current practitioner.

When the patient talks about other helpers, including her own parents, it is important for the practitioner to keep in mind not only that the patient is referring to him, but to think over what is in the material that the patient cannot discuss directly. Something about the love, hatred, or ambivalence is too embarrassing or shameful to be discussed in the open and the therapist has to keep this in mind as he relates to it.

> When Laura, a single woman in her early thirties, described in her third therapy session a female physician who was cold and withholding, her female therapist, Dr. M., soon realized that references to the physician were subtle ascriptions to herself. However, Dr. M. also recognized that it was too early to confront Laura with this, because the transference reactions were unconscious. Yet Dr. M. also was aware of the fact that if she did not relate to these negative feelings, Laura could act them out and quit treatment.
>
> In the fourth session, Dr. M. asked Laura if she had been able to share with that physician some of Laura's feelings toward her. When Laura told Dr. M. that she was frightened to share her negative feelings "toward almost anyone, particularly professionals," Dr. M. was able to say, "Perhaps it might be difficult and uncomfortable then to share your

criticisms of me." Though Laura turned several shades of red, hearing Dr. M.'s remark eventually enabled her to tell Dr. M. that at times she was "a bit cold and withholding." When Dr. M. told Laura that she was pleased Laura could share these reactions to her, the working alliance began to take form.

Almost any interaction that the patient describes has elements of the current transference to the therapist. In my own practice in which I have seen a lot of men and women who are therapists themselves, they have taught me that almost any reference to one of their patients is a reference to how they are feeling toward me. The following vignette relates to this.

Nat, an experienced clinician in his middle thirties, told me in his third session that he had just begun working with a patient who had a lot of difficulty beginning treatment. Nat told me that his patient's ambivalence was difficult for him to relate to. After I asked Nat to describe the patient's productions in detail, I said, "Beginning a therapeutic relationship can be tough." In response Nat asked, "Oh, is it tough for you to get started with me?" Then I responded, "Oh, is it tough for you to get started with me?" At this juncture we both laughed, but were able afterward to move ahead because we could discuss Nat's ambivalence toward me.

If the practitioner does not realize and accept that virtually every interpersonal interaction that the patient describes has implications for the current transference, he will have difficulty keeping the patient in treatment. This is particularly true when the patient is trying to discuss parts of the negative transference and is not being helped to do so.

AVOIDANCE OF THE COUNTERTRANSFERENCE

One of the greatest advances made in the last twenty years in psychotherapy is that mental health practitioners now accept that countertransference is as everpresent as is transference (Slakter 1987). If the therapist does not constantly study his feelings toward the patient, he can find himself becoming either too rejecting, too ingratiating, or a combination of these and other attitudes that are counterproductive.

Usually there is a correspondence between how the patient is responding to treatment and the therapist's countertransference. When the patient is reporting positive feelings toward the therapist and the therapy, she is probably picking up positive vibes from the therapist. The same is true of negative feelings that the patient reports about the therapy and therapist.

In the early phases of treatment, countertransference reactions are more difficult to detect. It usually takes a while before the therapist is aware of what he feels toward the patient. However, if he prolongs the sessions or shortens them, it is usually an indication that the therapist is not facing certain feelings toward the patient. Forgetting an appointment, wishing the session to be over, and not being able to concentrate are early signs of negative countertransference that have to be studied.

> When Dr. O, an experienced therapist, found himself extending the first three sessions with his patient Penelope, an attractive forty-year-old woman, Dr. O. decided to discuss this in supervision. He found that Penelope reminded him of an old girlfriend whom he occasionally wished he had married. Seeing Penelope in treatment was like a wish come true. However, Dr. O. had to work hard for several months in order to enable himself to treat Penelope rather than make her a girlfriend.

When the countertransference reactions are monitored well and the transference responses are well understood by patient and therapist, the honeymoon phase becomes a valuable experience for both. It serves as a useful contributor to a solid working alliance. But like all honeymoons, it comes to an end and the first treatment crisis sooner or later appears. We will discuss this challenging phase of treatment in the next chapter.

CHAPTER FOUR

The First Treatment Crisis: When Threats to Quit Treatment Are Common

No honeymoon lasts forever! Regardless of the intense and unambivalent passion that lovers can experience, harsh reality sooner or later intrudes and interpersonal conflict between them is inevitable. Just as the doting lover begins to recognize that her idealized man is not perfect but has limitations, patients in psychotherapy eventually have to face the fact that their therapists have flaws and cannot provide them with eternal bliss.

Confronting the fact that the perfect therapist, like the perfect mate, does not exist and therefore is not omnipotent, omniscient, or omnipresent is hardly ever a pleasant discovery. Most of the time it is a very disappointing event that arouses considerable resentment. The hostility of the patient in psychotherapy after the honeymoon is over is often so strong that it can lead to the premature ending of therapy. And this, of course, parallels the frequency of divorces that occur during the first year of marriage.

Similar to the newlywed who is insufficiently reassured, reaffirmed, and reinforced, many patients in psychotherapy want more than empathetic understanding. They get tired of continual catharsis, desiring instead to be told frequently that they are outstanding human beings who are very much admired and loved by the therapist. Most of the time they want to be his favorite and most idealized patient, as if they were a perfect mate.

Those of us who do marriage counseling note frequently a dimension of marital interaction that parallels therapeutic interaction. Many husbands and wives cannot tolerate for too long the pleasures and intimacies of a marital union. So too in psychotherapy, many patients become anxious if they are not censured when they express sexual or aggressive fantasies. They miss the punishment they think they deserve. And just as the honeymoon in marriage induces a regression in the partners, many patients during the honeymoon phase of therapy feel like little children. When little children become preoccupied with "the forbidden," they often provoke the punishment they believe they deserve. This is what many patients try to do after the honeymoon has lasted a while. They unconsciously want the therapist to berate them for their fantasied crimes and other subjective misdemeanors.

Another one of the characteristics of most marriages after they have endured for several months is that the mates resent the "lack of space" and the control and influence their partners exert. This inevitably happens in psychotherapy. Patients become annoyed that they must attend therapy sessions on a regular basis and often feel demeaned and derogated by the therapist's seeming power. This is what probably prompted the writer Lucy Freeman (1989) to describe her own personal therapy as being "The Beloved Prison."

Because experienced clinicians are aware of the fact that all human relationships contain elements of ambivalence, they become accustomed to being lauded and idealized at one moment and then castigated and berated at another. Conducting psychotherapy requires the practitioner to be comfortable with a range of emotions from patients that extends all the way from the epitome of love and admiration during the honeymoon phase of treatment to the most intense forms of hatred and derision during the first treatment crisis.

When patients end their honeymoons as their punitive superego reasserts itself and their id wishes become too frightening to them within a relationship that appears too intimate for them (Fine 1982), therapists become the recipients of all their anxiety and hostility. The merits of psychotherapy are questioned along with the practitioner's capabilities. Patients start to wonder if they are seeing the right therapist and/or are being treated with the right therapeutic modality. Maybe group therapy is more suitable than individual treatment? Possibly the frequency of the treatment should be lowered? And isn't the fee too high? Surely the hours could be more convenient? Couldn't the therapist say more? Offer some advice and/or reassurance? And just as newlyweds frequently contend they could find a better mate who is more giving, more understanding, and more sensitive, patients frequently aver that if they could find a different therapist, the chemistry in the patient–therapist interaction would be much more stimulating and more gratifying.

When a spouse castigates her partner, it is rarely easy for the partner to be completely understanding and unthreatened. Just as marriage partners become defensive under the impact of criticism and other direct and indirect attacks, many clinicians react similarly. It is not easy to neutrally and empathically respond to the patient's frequent tardiness, cancellations, or withholding of the fee. It can be upsetting to be told by the patient that the therapy is not helpful and maybe it should be terminated, and it can be humiliating to be contrasted with other therapists who guarantee better and faster therapeutic results.

One of the common errors of beginning clinicians when they are being attacked is to try immediately to show the patient that she is distorting the therapist and reacting negatively to him because of her unresolved problems. Although there is usually some distortion in every negative transference reaction, it usually takes most patients quite a while before they are ready to face that truth.

There are also those therapists who appear similar to masochistic spouses. They are always ready to take the blame for everything in order to secure the partner's love (Reik 1941). Therefore, they join their patients and berate themselves for their incompetent therapeutic behavior. They would rather demean themselves than face being abandoned by their patients, not realizing that their self-effacing and ingratiating behavior does not lessen the intensity or discomfort of the first treatment crisis.

The first treatment crisis, if not handled properly, can lead to the patient's quitting treatment. As the patient shows signs of negative transferential behavior coupled with an array of other provocative resistances, it is necessary for the therapist to listen carefully and empathically to her with a view toward understanding her and not toward "doing something." This is not a time for advice, reassurance, or environmental manipulation. It is a time for quiet listening and reflection.

In this chapter we will explore the various forms of behavior patients utilize to express their discomfort with the treatment crisis. We will focus primarily on the appropriate and inappropriate ways the therapist can respond to them.

VARIOUS EXPRESSIONS BY THE PATIENT OF THE FIRST TREATMENT CRISIS

Fixed Ideas

When human beings are uncomfortable with the feelings that have been induced by another person, they have a tendency to either avoid or attack the other person. Therefore, if dependency wishes, sexual yearnings, or aggressive fantasies aroused in the therapeutic situation cause anxiety for the patient then she is going to find a way to avoid or attack the therapist (Freud 1926, 1938, 1939). One way to maintain distance between the therapist and herself is to find something about him that may be real or fantasied and constantly condemn him for it. I remember when I first started doing therapy over forty-five years ago I was frequently told by patients that I was too young to be trusted with their lives. Today I'm frequently told that I'm too old to be trusted with their lives! I've been called "too Freudian" and "not Freudian enough." I've been experienced as too tall and too short. Some patients have felt I've been too concerned with sexual matters and some have felt I was completely asexual. Some have experienced me as too active while others have perceived me as too passive. Some have experienced me as emotionally and physically healthy while others have me crazy or dying. In working with patients during their first treatment crisis, I am often reminded of numerous songs whose refrains refer to being too young or too old, too rich or too poor, too this or too that. . . .

It is important for the practitioner to keep in mind when he is being criticized for one or more personal characteristics of his not just how valid and reliable the patient's perception is but, of perhaps even more importance, the therapist should remind himself that the patient has a wish to keep a distance from the therapist and weaken his influence. If the patient is extremely threatened by emerging feelings such as homosexual desires, intense competition, or powerful dependency longings, she may work hard to find sufficient justification to prove that the therapist is totally incompetent and possibly should be removed from the profession.

Reuben Fine (1982) relates a story of his mentor, the eminent psychoanalyst Theodor Reik. Apparently Reik had a patient who said to him, "You are not Theodor Reik." The patient was so convinced that Reik was an impostor that he wrote to the University of Vienna where Reik had obtained his doctorate. The officials could not verify that Reik graduated from the university because the records were lost during World War II. Triumphantly the patient said, "That proves my case" and left treatment, carrying on a long vendetta regarding Reik's qualifications.

Reik's story is very instructive. It reveals that when a patient is discharging fury at a therapist during a treatment crisis, she appears very similar to a misunderstood, frustrated, and unloved spouse. Through the expression of her prolonged and intense hatred, she is also revealing how very much involved she is with her partner. If the dissatisfied spouse or unhappy patient were not feeling a lot of mixed feelings toward the marital or therapy partner, she would just leave. Her indignation, like Theodor Reik's patient's, shows that she is "protesting too much."

Frustration of honeymoon fantasies leaves the patient furious. She should be loved always and must have constant love that is available to her pronto. She is entitled to it. Some patients feel that to be adored by the therapist is a right. Many patients during their first treatment crisis have been described by Shakespeare in *Richard II*: "Sweet love, I see, changing his property/Turns to the sourest and most deadly hate."

Because of the intense and complex emotions aroused during the first treatment crisis, it becomes clear that no series of questions, clarifying remarks, or interpretations is going to change the patient's hostile stance. As a matter of fact, if the therapist has too much to say, the patient will perceive his remarks as argumentative and will gladly participate in an ongoing verbal battle.

When Zelda, a married woman in her forties, had been in treatment with Dr. Y. for about four months, she began to find fault with him. She told him that his clothes were drab, his office decor was inappropriate, and his mannerisms were somewhat effeminate. Not seeing that Zelda was reacting to the disappointment that she was experiencing because many of her sexual and dependency longings were not being gratified, and unaware of how angry he was as he went from "a perfect man" to "a lowly one" in Zelda's eyes, Dr. Y. made a long interpretation. He told Zelda she was eager to castrate him because he reminded her of her father, who was not available to her. He also spoke of her unresolved "penis envy" and other "conflicts."

Zelda responded to Dr. Y.'s "interpretations" with much anger and told him that he was envious of Zelda's "assertive capacities" and other "assets." Dr. Y., in turn, had other "interpretations" to make which succeeded in getting Zelda even more furious. After about two months of vindictive interchanges, Zelda quit treatment.

What is important to keep in mind about the above case illustration of Zelda and Dr. Y. is that almost everything they had to say about each other was essentially true. However, it was said in anger. One of the important lessons that we learn from this vignette is that if the therapist responds with anger to the patient's anger, it only begets more anger until a battle royal ensues. If the issues that provoked the battle are not confronted, treatment usually ends prematurely.

Whenever a patient criticizes a therapist, the therapist must give the criticism a fair and long hearing without interrupting the patient with comments. In effect, the therapist should try to monitor his hurt and anger and try to use it to understand the patient better. He can help the patient by listening to her complaints and try to see what motivates her attacks.

York, a single man in his late twenties, was in therapy with Ms. W. Treatment had been going well for the first three months but then York started to come late for sessions, had little to say in the sessions, and found reasons to stay away from several of them. When Ms. W. suggested to York that perhaps his lateness, absences, and limited participation in the sessions could be a reflection of some of his dissatisfaction with her, York at first denied this possibility and changed the subject. However, when Ms. W. later pointed out that he seemed to feel uncomfortable criticizing her, York was eventually able to express some of his frustrations with the treatment.

York told Ms. W. that the main reason he found meeting with her to be difficult for him is that she was "a cold person." His life experience had taught him that cold people couldn't be trusted in human relationships and therefore York had been considering going to another therapist. As a matter of fact he had a consultation with another therapist a few days ago and the therapist told York that he was quite sure he could help York more than he was being helped by Ms. W.

As Ms. W. quietly studied her reactions to York's comments and actions, she realized how angry and hurt she felt. She had been trying her best to be an attentive, empathetic therapist and instead of being appreciated, was being rejected. Furthermore, Ms. W. had been enjoying the first few months of her work with York and after being elevated to a lofty position, she was feeling like the scum of the earth, and it hurt.

As Ms. W. studied her reactions to York, she realized that a good part of what she was feeling, York must have wanted her to feel (Maroda 1994). She knew she wasn't feeling cold toward York and had enjoyed the mutual warmth that seemed to be present heretofore. Further, Ms. W. recalled how much York had resented "eager" women like his mother and older sister who wanted to "manipulate" him.

Although Ms. W. knew that York was far away from recognizing his own need for distance, she nonetheless had to help York eventually get in touch with it. Consequently, she asked York if he thought he might feel more comfortable working with a man and that perhaps that may have influenced his seeking out a male therapist for a consultation. This question helped York. He told Ms. W. that he was convinced "women tried to get into your skin" and "get all your feelings, while men didn't." Furthermore, he likened Ms. W. to his mother, "who wanted too much" of him.

As York could vent his irritation with Ms. W. for being a controlling and intrusive woman like his mother and saw that Ms. W. warmly listened to him without saying very much, York's attacks diminished and he was able by the eighth month of therapy to acknowledge how "desperately afraid" he was of an intimate relationship with a woman.

Love frequently turns to hate after the honeymoon is over (Gabbard 1996) but, as I've already suggested, the reasons for the switch differ from patient to patient. In York's case, he was becoming frightened of the warmth and intimacy he was feeling toward his therapist. In other situations, the patient may be feeling competitive and want to defeat the therapist, or she may become frightened of her dependency or aggression. It is the practitioner's job to ferret out what is disturbing the patient and sometimes it takes many sessions until the therapist can be sure of what is going on.

Veronica, in her late teens, was being seen in therapy for many psychosomatic ailments such as gastrointestinal problems, migraine headaches, and insomnia. Her therapist, Mr. U., was able to help her diminish her symptoms by enlisting her cooperation in discharging many aggressive fantasies toward her mother. According to Veronica, her mother watched her behavior "like a hawk" and Veronica resented it very much.

With her symptomatology reduced by the fourth month of treatment, Veronica was feeling very positive toward her therapy and Mr. U. In the next several weeks she spent much of her time talking about the growth in her self-confidence and self-esteem, as well as her ability to be more assertive.

However, from a position of gratitude and elation, Veronica began suddenly to question the wisdom of being in therapy. She had many friends who had been in treatment and had found their therapists to be unhelpful and incompetent.

Although Mr. U. knew that Veronica was feeling uncomfortable about something in their relationship, he didn't know what it was. Inquiries on his part yielded next to nothing. As Mr. U. was feeling helpless without much hope, Veronica helped him by referring to a former teacher who "smiled arrogantly all the time and felt too smug." He knew this had to do with him because other patients and colleagues had described him this way on occasion. When he suggested to Veronica that maybe he appeared arrogant with his smile, Veronica denied this. However, when Mr. U. told Veronica that he had been experienced this way by others in the past, it helped her.

Veronica spent much time telling Mr. U. that his "realistic" expression was one of "haughtiness" and that, while she knew he "couldn't cut it out right away," she "hated" it. As Veronica noted that Mr. U. did not react defensively but acknowledged that his demeanor could be irritating, Veronica felt much less hostile and stayed in treatment. She eventually could tell Mr. U. that his "arrogant smiling" reminded her of her father's "smugness" and that she frequently felt demeaned by him.

Alibis

Although most patients are not much aware of what is activating their first treatment crisis, there are some patients who consciously use alibis to express their resentment toward and discomfort with the treatment situation. Rather than talking about what upsets them about the therapy and the therapist, they find reasons to try to stay uninvolved.

Patients can complain that the scheduled sessions are becoming too inconvenient, that the fee is draining, or that the travel is too expensive and time-consuming. The reason these patients are difficult to work with is that most of the time the therapist knows the patient is using alibis but can't confront her with her manipulations; she would deny them.

The main clue to the patient's using alibis is her affect. She becomes indignant about the schedule, furious about the fee, contemptuous about the office decor, all of which seriously interferes with her comfort in the therapeutic situation. There is only a thinly veiled hostility toward the practitioner, but enough to make it clear that the therapy poses a threat to the patient.

More often than not the patient who uses alibis induces strong countertransference reactions in the therapist. The reason for this is that few practitioners like to be manipulated and this is precisely what the patient is trying to do: deceive the therapist. In effect, the patient is doing the opposite of what we usually want from our therapeutic partner. Instead of talking about what she feels and thinks and then trying to understand it, this individual moves away from being an introspective patient with feelings; this usually frustrates us.

When a patient moves far away from exploring herself, we can infer how terribly dangerous the therapeutic situation is for her. She is worried that her dependency might make her a compliant but helpless and symbiotic child. She fears that cooperation with the therapist will make her a slave, and she is apprehensive that warm and sexual feelings toward the therapist may lead to some acting out.

If the therapist can remind himself that the alibiing patient is a very frightened and timid person, his punctured narcissism usually recedes and the negative countertransference becomes less powerful. I have found that once I am able to acknowledge and then monitor my angry feelings toward the alibiing patient and don't feel that my status as a therapist is in as much jeopardy, I can deal with the alibi or alibis with more finesse.

I have come to the conclusion that during the first treatment crisis the therapist should *not* confront the patient with the fact that she is alibiing. Rather, I believe the practitioner should try his best to respond to the alibi as something valid and then observe what the patient does as she is accepted for what she presents. For example, when the patient tells me during the first treatment crisis that the scheduled time is inconvenient, I try to explore with her what makes the time inconvenient and what would be a better time for her. Or, if the patient points out that she is unable to pay the current fee, I try to discuss with her what her financial situation is and what she thinks she can afford.

Many clinicians are reluctant to take the patient who is alibiing at face value because they worry they will be controlled, overpowered, or demeaned. They get concerned about the patient's destroying the therapeutic frame and not respecting the boundaries of treatment. The reason for this is that the practitioner thinks that if he discusses with the patient what she does not like about the appointment time and how she would like it improved he is under some obligation to make a switch and keep making switches.

What most clinicians learn is that when they don't get into an argument or power struggle with the patient over her alibis, but attempt to understand what is going on in the patient's psychic life, the alibi loses its potency and the psychic truth tends to emerge.

> Tom, a 19-year-old student, who was in therapy because he was about to be flunked out of college, had come to his appointments regularly for about three months. During this time, he voiced a great deal of resentment toward teachers and peers and was also able to talk about missing home.

Tom's catharses helped him do better in his courses and it was clear that he was growing fond of his female therapist, Ms. S.

Toward the end of his fourth month of treatment, Tom told Ms. S. that he would have to reduce the frequency of his sessions from twice a week to once a week because he had to take a part-time job. The reason he needed to take a job was because he knew his parents did not like paying so much money for his college tuition, his therapy, and his other expenses.

As Ms. S. listened to Tom, she felt that he was using several alibis at once. She was quite sure that his parents were not putting pressure on him to work nor were they complaining about financing Tom's education either. However, after she got on top of her own anger and realized that Tom was trying to push her away because he was frightened of the growing intimacy between them, she asked Tom which day he was working: maybe they could change that appointment? After some hesitancy, Tom pointed out that he did not know his working hours, but when Ms. S. later asked about the job, it turned out he had not yet been hired.

When Tom saw that Ms. S. did not question the veracity of his statements but just wanted to understand what was happening regarding the job, Tom was able to point out that he was "finding the therapy a bit of a drag." Then Ms. S. could say, "Perhaps we can talk about what you don't like about seeing me twice a week?"

Tom eventually was able to discuss with Ms. S. how much he feared his growing dependency on her and how she was becoming a "mother figure" who could control his life too much. Once Tom could face his dependent transference toward Ms. S., he did not need his alibis anymore.

What is important for the clinician constantly to keep in mind is that the patient who uses alibis is frightened of the truth. To face the truth for this patient is to face feelings that pose a danger, and it is the danger that we want to help the patient discuss with us. As we saw with Tom in the case above, when he could discharge his concerns about depending on a mother figure he did not need to use alibis as a defense as much.

The Treatment Doesn't Work!

In a book written in 1923 entitled *The Ego and the Id*, Sigmund Freud discussed the *negative therapeutic reaction*. Freud was referring to the responses of the patient who seems to accept all of the therapist's interpretations and other interventions, but does not get better; sometimes she gets worse. Freud attributed this phenomenon to the patient's punitive superego, which does not permit her to enjoy the fruits of therapeutic success.

As clinicians after Freud have examined the negative therapeutic reaction more closely, they have been able to determine that at its core is the patient's unconscious wish to defeat the therapist. Although the patient is not overtly hostile, there is a part of her that experiences the therapist as a narcissistic, arrogant, and insensitive parent who should not feel pleased with himself for achieving good therapeutic results. Instead, the therapist should suffer the way the patient has suffered heretofore, even if that means that the patient does not make any therapeutic progress.

Very often the negative therapeutic reaction is at its height during the first treatment crisis. The reason for this is that the patient, after reflecting on the honeymoon with her therapist, resents the power and control he has over her. To demonstrate that the therapist is really unimportant, the patient unconsciously destroys the therapist's positive impact.

Like the rebellious child who does not overtly challenge her parents or other figures of authority, but secretly defeats them by her seeming inability to be toilet-trained, read, write, or adapt to other requirements, the patient with the negative therapeutic reaction fights the therapist's objectives. If the patient thinks that the therapist is eager to see symptoms removed, the patient will keep saying, "I don't know why my migraine headaches, stomach pains, and ulcer keep returning ." Or, if the patient believes that the therapist would like to see her marital problems decrease in severity, for some strange reason the marital conflicts become exacerbated.

Inasmuch as this type of patient we are discussing is most frustrating to the therapist, he is inclined to tell the patient how she is sabotaging the therapy. And because the patient is so negativistic, she will probably insist that she is trying her best to be cooperative. Further, if one overlooks unconscious motivation, the patient is quite sincere in her proclamations.

I have found that the most productive way to deal with the patient with a negative therapeutic reaction is that, when the therapist is criticized, he should be willing initially to take some responsibility for the treatment not working. Without consciously realizing it, when she sees that the therapist blames himself the negativistic patient wants to oppose the therapist and does so by focusing more on herself and her own motives. What the practitioner has to keep in mind, if he elects to focus on his own shortcomings, is when the patient appears cooperative and insightful he cannot and should not exude too much pleasure. If he does, the patient will work harder to defeat him.

A married woman in her mid-thirties, Ruth was in treatment with Dr. P., a male therapist, because of severe sexual inhibitions. After a six-month honeymoon in which she could for the first time in her adult life experience sexual pleasure, Ruth slowly began to return to her former ways of coping. She had increased the frequency of her sessions during the honeymoon to three times a week; now, Ruth wanted to return to once a week. During the honeymoon phase of treatment she had many fewer arguments with her husband; now, she was having more than ever before. Almost every dimension of her life was deteriorating and Ruth kept telling Dr. P. that she was "a hopeless, helpless, failed case."

Dr. P., an experienced clinician, recognized that Ruth was undergoing a negative therapeutic reaction and felt that, though it would take a long time, he wanted to help Ruth feel her wish to destroy him and the therapy.

As he listened to Ruth talk on and on about her lack of improvement, he realized that unconsciously Ruth was getting quite a bit of gratification out of it. Although he knew that the last thing in the world he could say was that Ruth was a defeater, he did say to her, "It's quite clear that I haven't been helping you. I think we should try to figure out what I've been doing wrong!"

Ruth protested and told Dr. P. she was a "hopeless case." When Dr. P. told Ruth that he thought maybe he was a "hopeless therapist," Ruth became indignant and informed Dr. P. that his self-abnegating attitude was very frustrating. She further told him that he should feel more self-confident and not so weak. Dr. P., realizing that Ruth was already beginning to bring out some of her rage through her criticisms of him, asked for more information from her about his lack of confidence. However, Ruth, sensing that this is what Dr. P. wanted to learn more about, began to talk about herself.

Ruth told Dr. P. that in many ways she felt she was back in the third grade, when she was "a failing student." At the time she was in the third grade, just like the present, she was trying her best to do well, but she kept floundering. When Dr. P. asked Ruth what she felt in the third grade classroom that was similar to what she felt in his office, Ruth spontaneously said, "We're not with each other; we're against each other."

Dr. P. tried his best to monitor his enthusiasm as Ruth got more in touch with her rebelliousness and sadism. As she talked more about her defiance, her life improved a great deal, but it was close to a year before Dr. P. felt that he could focus with Ruth on her fight with him and her wish to defeat him.

The negative therapeutic reaction, like most phenomena, occurs at various times throughout the entire treatment.

Few patients are exempt from the wish to seek revenge toward their parents; consequently, few therapists are exempt from being devalued and demeaned by the patient. The most helpful way to resolve the negative therapeutic reaction is for the practitioner to openly question himself and acknowledge that he may be doing something that is interfering with therapeutic progress. Most negativistic patients want to prove him wrong and usually start to examine themselves.

The Flight into Health

In contrast to the negative therapeutic reaction, where the patient doesn't improve or gets worse, the flight into health is a mechanism whereby the patient, in fear of facing herself, unconsciously arranges to give up her symptoms (Sandler et al. 1973). For some patients the threat that therapy is to their psychic equilibrium is so great they try to justify their wish to terminate treatment by pointing out that their conflicts have disappeared. For these patients, their worry that their therapy may lead to a divorce from their spouses, a reevaluation of their job situation, or some other disruption to their current modus vivendi can motivate them to relinquish the primary and secondary gains they derive from their symptoms and from their other neurotic conflicts.

The flight into health should be viewed as a resistance to self-understanding. The patient, rather than face the dynamics of her fights with her husband or with others, gives up the fights and, of course, concomitantly wants to give up treatment. I recall working with a man who quickly gave up twenty years of stuttering in order to avoid facing his acute separation anxiety (Strean 1998). I also recall treating a woman who, rather than face her homosexuality, impulsively got married and quit therapy.

As implied, when a patient flees into health we realize that the behavior is a defense that must be respected, rather than a piece of behavior that can be overlooked or criticized. Like other resistances, when the practitioner does not fight the patient's unwillingness to remain in therapy, the patient usually begins to examine herself and frequently stays in treatment.

> Nate, a married man in his fifties, was in treatment with Dr. O., a female therapist who was about Nate's age. Nate sought treatment because he felt very depressed, because his wife was continuously criticizing him and rejecting him.
>
> In the therapeutic situation, Nate blossomed. He told Dr. O. that "for the first time in my life" he was with a woman who tried to understand him rather than judge him, support him rather than undermine him. By the fourth month of treatment, Nate's depression had lifted, he became more assertive at home and work, where he was an accountant, and found himself feeling more loving toward his children and friends.
>
> While Nate was enjoying a prolonged honeymoon with Dr. O., he began to have some dreams that created enormous conflict for him. In them he was leaving his wife and going off with Dr. O. as his partner. These dreams aroused much anxiety for Nate, since his hostility toward his wife frightened him and his libidinal fantasies toward Dr. O. stirred up much guilt.

In contrast to his openness and spontaneity in his earlier therapy sessions, Nate began to become more and more inhibited. Attempts by Dr. O. to explore this with him were resisted. In his sixth month of treatment, Nate pointed out that his relationship with his wife was much better, he was more assertive and she was more accepting, and it was now time to end therapy.

Although Dr. O. realized that Nate's behavior was a flight into health and that he was trying to avoid facing his hostility toward his wife and his sexual feelings toward her, Dr. O. took Nate's wish to quit treatment seriously.

Dr. O. asked Nate when he was planning to end treatment with her. Nate was nonplussed and blurted out, "I didn't think you'd take me so seriously!" As Dr. O. tried to explore his reaction, Nate said he was always ready to "be put down by a woman" when he "stands up."

Because Dr. O. did not argue with Nate but accepted his wish to quit treatment as something to be seriously discussed, Nate could reveal his castration anxiety as he related to a woman. Feeling safe with Dr. O., he could go on to examine his fears around sex and aggression.

It is important to keep in mind constantly when working with a patient who is exhibiting a flight into health that the flight is a device utilized to protect her against danger. Therefore, the practitioner should not challenge the wish to quit treatment until some of the patient's motives are clearer to both of them. When the patient appears to feel a little safer to reveal some of her anxiety, then the therapist can feel safer to clarify and interpret some of it.

When Family and Friends Oppose the Therapy

Regardless of a practitioner's theoretical predilections or preferred therapeutic modality, he soon becomes aware of an
unalterable fact, namely, some of the patient's family and
friends oppose her being in therapy (Ackerman 1958). There
are usually many reasons why this occurs. First and foremost,
family and friends fear losing the patient's love, and worry
that the attachment to the patient may be severed as she
attaches herself to the therapist and loves him. Secondly,
as the patient modifies her behavior and becomes more
assertive, more spontaneous, more loving, and less masochistic, those in her social orbit may not find her modified
behavior as compatible with their current modus vivendi.
Finally, it is quite possible that the patient may withdraw
cathexes from family and friends as her own autonomy becomes strengthened.

One major way family and friends deal with the anxiety
induced by the patient's involvement with her therapy and
her therapist is to criticize the treatment. If the patient is
upset by the negative comments of her friends and family,
she will probably bring these comments to treatment and see
what the therapist will do with them.

Over the years I have learned that even if the patient
condemns the negative comments about the therapist and
therapy, a part of her believes them or is using them to but-
tress a resistance. I have also learned that one of the most
common counterresistances of clinicians when patients report an outsider's criticism of the therapy is to try to join with
the patient and rebut the criticisms. This stance, obviously,

does not lead to productive therapy; on the contrary, it retards it.

If the practitioner keeps in mind that, when a patient says the spouse is doubting whether the therapy can help her, the patient has her own doubts, he will be less inclined to knock the spouse and/or defend himself. Rather, he will try to conduct himself in a way that facilitates the patient's expression of doubt and resentment about the therapy and therapist.

One of the best ways to help the patient eventually get in touch with the notion that when she quotes others she is really talking about herself is to ask her how she felt when the spouse (or other person) was critical of the therapist and/or the therapy. Occasionally the patient will report what she did say to those who attacked the therapist, and examination of the feelings that generated the retorts will usually be revealing to the therapist and eventually to the patient.

> Mary, in her early forties, was in intensive treatment three times a week with Dr. L., a male therapist. Prior to her therapy with Dr. L., Mary had seen several other therapists without much success. She had been very upset about her inability to achieve sustained relationships with men and was equally upset with the therapists who were not able to help her.
>
> Although Mary seemed to feel quite positive toward Dr. L. during the first several months of treatment, Dr. L. knew that sooner or later Mary's latent hostility toward men would have to emerge in her transference toward him.

Dr. L.'s expectations seemed to be validated when Mary mentioned that at a recent party she attended, several of the people had negative things to say about Dr. L. A couple of them knew him as a teacher and felt he was too "dogmatic" and some knew him as an author and contended that he was too "superficial."

In her sessions with Dr. L., Mary vehemently denounced Dr. L.'s detractors and proudly declared that she defended him when he was attacked. As Dr. L. listened carefully to Mary, he said to himself, "The lady doth protest too much." As he studied his feelings further, he eventually asked Mary, "What did it feel like to hear your therapist being attacked?" Mary spontaneously said, "Awful. It's a reflection on me. It means that I haven't *chosen* a competent person. I'm sort of in the position of a wife or fiancee hearing her man being knocked. It's as if a part of me is defective."

Inasmuch as Mary had a lot of trouble *choosing* men in her social life, Dr. L. knew that what was currently transpiring in the transference was crucial. Therefore, he was very mindful of how he would use himself in the treatment crisis that was just beginning. He asked Mary, "How does it feel to have a therapist who may be defective?" With this question, Mary's latent hostility came to the fore. She went on a rampage, berating Dr. L. for "being defective" and said she was always "ending up with men who had no balls."

After Mary spent several sessions bemoaning her fate and lamenting how she always ended up with losers, Dr. L. was able to make the interpretation that Mary had an unconscious wish to be with a loser. Although Mary fought

Dr. L.'s interpretation for some time, she was able to say in the eighth month of treatment, "There's too much evidence to support it. I guess it makes me feel stronger to have men weaker."

If the clinician keeps in mind that the patient's references to others and what they have to say about therapy and the therapist is a disguised message from the patient, he will be in a more secure position to help the patient resolve the first treatment crisis.

It should also be noted that anything the patient repeats about therapy and therapists that she hears from others is an indirect, albeit muffled, statement to the therapist. This also applies to patients who have difficulty stating compliments and who will quote others who say something positive about the therapist or therapy. This alerts the therapist to help the patient deal with the resistances against verbalizing compliments, just as negative statements from the outside alert the therapist to deal with the resistances of his patient against verbalizing resentments.

Shifting the Modality

One of the more obvious signs of an impending treatment crisis is the patient's wish to change the treatment modality. If the therapist accepts the notion that every request of a patient's should be explored, he will usually find out upon exploration that a request to drop a session of individual therapy and go into group therapy, or one that recommends that conjoint marital counseling should be added to or replace individual treatment, is an expression of resistance. While not questioning the efficacy of any specific therapeutic modality, we can say, however, that whenever the patient wants to modify the therapeutic modality in which she is currently involved, we can assume she is uncomfortable with her current therapy.

Usually when a therapist complies with the patient's request and shifts to a different therapeutic modality or initiates adding or shifting to another one, he, too, is uncomfortable with the present arrangement. Practitioners' reasons for changing the modality are usually similar to those of the patient. For example, if the therapist is uncomfortable treating a patient in individual therapy who has marital problems, rather than explore his discomfort, he can arrange for the patient to be seen with the spouse in conjoint marital counseling. Similarly, if the therapist is not resolving his counterresistances as he does conjoint marital counseling, he can recommend individual treatment.

Particularly in this day and age, when there is a plethora of treatment modalities available, it is easy to justify modifying the current modality in order to help the patient. Yet any time a practitioner wants to modify the modality, upon self-examination he will usually ascertain that he is experiencing discomfort with the patient. The patient's chronic hostility, demands, sexual interests, devaluation of the therapist, or a combination thereof are motivating his desire to switch.

> Jerry, in his early forties, was in treatment with Dr. K., a male therapist. Jerry had come to see Dr. K. because he was very upset about the fact this his wife was planning to

leave him. When Jerry acquiesced to going into therapy, his wife said she'd "stay around for a while and see if there are any changes."

In the therapy, Dr. K. immediately tried to help Jerry become a more cooperative husband by suggesting that he help his wife more with domestic chores and spend more time with the children. When this didn't have any appreciable effect on the marital relationship, Dr. K. tried to help Jerry become more assertive. This brought Jerry and his wife into more overt conflict and, therefore, Dr. K. recommended conjoint marital counseling.

In the conjoint counseling, the arguments grew, so Dr. K. tried to see Jerry and his wife individually. Soon after this, each of them terminated treatment and went to two separate therapists.

In this case, we see a very common occurrence in psychotherapy. Dr. K. was overidentified with his patient and therefore, to help preserve Jerry's marriage (which would be equivalent psychologically to making a desperate stab to save his own marriage), he tried to influence him to be compliant. When this didn't please Jerry's wife, Dr. K., in his overidentification, got angry at the wife and encouraged Jerry to retaliate. Dr. K.'s feelings of helplessness and anxiety grew stronger as he worked with Jerry, and because he never faced his feelings, his patient as well as the patient's wife, left him. Had Dr. K. been more self-aware, he would have been able to help Jerry face his own sadomasochism and see how he was turning himself into a son rather than be a husband.

COMMON ERRORS OF THERAPISTS DURING THE FIRST TREATMENT CRISIS: A SUMMARY

In this section we will briefly summarize the errors that practitioners frequently make during the first treatment crisis. If the practitioner understands better the whys and wherefores of his errors, he is less apt to repeat them in future crises with the patient and will feel more secure with future patients when having to deal with them in the same situation.

Virtually all of the errors listed below have been alluded to throughout this chapter.

1. Resisting Resistance

Therapists, like all honeymooners, do not like to face reality. Hence, they can be reluctant to face the fact that their patient is no longer passionately in love with them. Therefore, they can ignore lateness, absences, increased symptomatology, and wishes of the patient to change treatment modality, and not see them as signs of a growing negative transference.

2. Coping with the Patient's Anger with Angry Interventions

When a patient's anger toward the therapist and her devaluation of the therapist and the treatment is threatening to the therapist, he can handle his anger by making hostile interpretations and confrontations. Often statements about the patient's "penis envy," "wish to castrate," or "competition" with the therapist are thinly disguised accusations that are designed to weaken the patient and make her appear less threatening to him.

3. Accepting the Patient's Criticisms as Completely Valid

When the therapist has strong wishes to be loved by the patient and therefore cannot deal with her hostility, he may go out of his way to take all of the patient's complaints as legitimate. Then, he may switch the treatment modality if the patient requests it and gratify any request without sufficiently exploring it. In effect, the therapist becomes like a masochistic spouse who must always be a servant.

4. Giving Advice and Intervening in the Patient's Life

During the first treatment crisis, the patient's negative transference may be defended against by feelings of helplessness. Not recognizing the patient's inability to deal with her life as a function of her growing dissatisfaction with treatment, the therapist mistakenly sees members of the patient's family, calls her doctor, meets with her lawyer, or gives all kinds of advice. The patient's neurotic dependency increases and her negative transference goes unexplored.

5. Challenging or Refuting the Patient's Negative Comments about Treatment

When a patient finds fault with the treatment or with the practitioner, the therapy is never helped by telling the patient she is wrong. Rather, the patient needs to express her complaints and voice her anger. It is only after doing so that she might be willing to explore herself.

6. Showing Too Much Enthusiasm with Results

In order to do effective therapy, the therapist has to provide an environment in which the patient gains increasing security in saying everything she feels and thinks. If the therapist is too pleased with the therapeutic results, the patient feels increasingly pressured to produce for him. Further, if the therapist becomes too happy, the competition of the patient becomes aroused and then she will try to make him miserable. One sure way is to get worse and another is to leave or threaten to leave treatment.

Mishandling of Situational Crises and the Patient's Readiness to Quit Treatment

Assuming that the first treatment crisis has been resolved, the patient will then form a therapeutic alliance (Greenson 1967) with the therapist and use his healthy ego functions, together with the therapist's, to try to understand and master the conflicts in the patient's life. Having weathered the storms of the first treatment crisis with the concomitant intensification of the therapeutic alliance, patient and therapist are now better equipped to deal with the inevitable crises that are bound to occur during the rest of the treatment process.

I have often noted that, if the first treatment crisis has been mastered well, the patient becomes more secure and more confident as he attempts to resolve crises with his spouse, children, colleagues, and friends. Of equal importance, he becomes less frightened to look at himself and more courageously faces his fantasies, his guilts, his dreams, and his past.

Yet, regardless of the patient's growth and despite his ego functions that work well, all patients continue to resist the treatment process. One of the most common resistances that patients utilize is to overemphasize reality. If the patient has marital conflicts, he will have a strong tendency to use his sessions to describe his altercations with his wife and hope that the therapist will agree with him that his wife is the immature member of the marital union and can't relate well to him. Similarly, if the patient is a single person and is unsuccessful in finding a mate, he, too, will use many of his sessions to describe his unsuccessful pursuits, and blame the culture, the city he lives in, or the women for his unhappy plight.

Every patient, to some extent, prefers to see himself as a victim of circumstance rather than the editor-in-chief of his life's problems. Parents blame children for their interpersonal difficulties and vice versa. Bosses and their subordinates do the same thing. And, if the patient does not find another person in his social orbit to blame for his difficulties, he might focus on his poor looks, malformed body, small penis, or underdeveloped intelligence. Possibly he is the victim of sexism, racism, or some other form of discrimination, but he's definitely a victimized soul who does not deserve to be blamed for his sad life. His parents are; his spouse is; his culture is!

Even when patients blame themselves, their masochistic orgies (Fine 1982) often mask a wish for the listener to attack those whom the patient really believes are the source of his maladies. As Reik (1941) has poignantly described, the masochistic patient looks like a lamb but is really a wolf!

One of the great contributions of psychodynamic psychotherapy (Freud 1939) is the notion that nothing happens by chance. Whom we marry, how we relate to our children, the type of interactions we have with our colleagues and friends, how we view ourselves and others are a function of our inner life, which is composed of fantasies, superego commands, memories, and a host of other idiosyncratic variables.

Psychodynamic psychotherapy contends that, for a patient to improve his psychosexual functioning and lead a happier life, he must face his instinctual wishes, defensive operations, and superego introjects.

One of the reasons that effective therapy takes some time and often requires the patient to have frequent sessions is that he has such a tendency not to face himself, but would rather analyze and hypothesize about others instead. In effect, his resistances need a lot of attention (Strean 1990).

Just as the patient's major resistance can be an overemphasis on reality, I have found that the major counter-resistance of therapists can be their tendency to focus too much on reality and not nearly enough on the patient's fantasies, dream life, and other internal variables. This is why a lot of therapy is not very successful. The patient in a marital struggle, for example, is not sufficiently helped to understand why he sought out the wife he married and what gratifications and protections his marital disputes offer him (Strean 1996a). The unattached patient who consciously abhors his single life is not sufficiently confronted by the therapist with what he is doing to sustain this single status (Strean 1995a). The same can be said about the treatment of many parents, who are given too much advice about childrearing and insufficient information about what gratifications and protections their children's symptoms provide for them.

Inasmuch as I am very convinced that one of the major factors in patient dropout and in other unsuccessful therapy is the patient's and therapist's overemphasis on reality—on situational factors—to the detriment of exploring the patient's inner life, which accounts for much of his maladaptive functioning, this chapter is an attempt to redress this continuing problem in psychotherapeutic practice. I would like to note parenthetically that managed care, with its emphasis on short-term treatment and its almost exclusive focus on reality, would not be such a dominant force on the contemporary psychotherapeutic scene if clinicians had more conviction that the patient's inner life is the engine that generates his behavior and that this is what needs our undivided therapeutic attention.

In this chapter I would like to focus on the most common situational factors that are presented to clinicians. In my discussion I want to demonstrate what internal variables account for the patient's situational distress and, of equal importance, how the therapist can help and not help the patient resolve the realistic problems he brings to us.

I will, in this chapter, discuss in detail marital conflict, parent–child problems, some of the conflicts of the unattached patient, work problems, gender, racial, and religious difficulties, and issues that patients bring in regarding their appearance and body image. As suggested, of crucial importance, we will also discuss in detail the therapist's use of herself as she tries to help the patient resolve his situational conflicts.

MARITAL CONFLICTS

Certainly in mental health treatment centers and social agencies, and perhaps in private practice as well, the modal patient is one who is unhappily married and wants the therapist to fix his marriage or help him get a divorce. This patient is full of complaints about the spouse. She is, according to the patient, too demanding, too critical, insufficiently sensitive, and not sexually satisfying. The patient may give some lip service to how he contributes to the marital dysfunctioning but most of his time in therapy is spent lamenting his condition.

One of the important discoveries made through the study of marital conflict is that every chronic marital complaint is an unconscious wish (Strean 1996a). The husband who chronically complains that his wife is cold and asexual unconsciously wants such a wife. A warm and sexual wife would frighten him. Consequently, one of the reasons he constantly complains about his marital partner is that he knows on some level that his complaints won't bring her closer. Similarly, the wife who chronically complains that her husband is weak and passive unconsciously wants such a man. A strong, assertive man would scare her, and that is one of the reasons she constantly derides him. If she praised him and he emerged as more self-confident it would arouse enormous anxiety in her.

How do we know that the chronic marital complaint is an unconscious wish? Because if the therapist does not take sides in the marital conflict but instead helps the patient explore his fantasies, conflicts, and history, he will begin to relate to the therapist the same way he relates to his spouse. If the spouse is experienced as depriving and hostile, sooner or later the therapist will be perceived similarly. This, of course, will take place only if the therapist maintains her neutrality and helps the patient express what is really on his mind.

One of the reasons many patients are not sufficiently helped with their marital conflicts is that their therapists do not view their complaints as emanating largely from within. Thus, they attempt to help their patients behave in such a way that will change their partners' behaviors. This hardly ever works! If a husband can't stand his wife's overeating, for example, and the therapist tries to help him change his wife's behavior, the patient may get worse because the gratifications and protections he derives from his wife's overeating are frustrated. Unless the patient understands what unconscious factors are at work that make him focus constantly on his wife's eating, his wish to deride her will continue and he will be very anxious without criticizing her constantly.

Agnes, a married woman in her early thirties, had been in therapy with Dr. B., a male therapist, in order to try to resolve some of her marital conflicts. She incessantly told Dr. B. that her husband, Charlie, was asexual, unromantic, weak, passive, and insensitive. Dr. B. tried to help Agnes praise Charlie instead of criticizing him so much. Most of the time Agnes opposed Dr. B.'s suggestions, and when she tried on occasion to implement them, Charlie was unresponsive. Shortly after Dr. B. suggested to Agnes that she try "a trial separation," Agnes left treatment.

A couple of months later Agnes went into treatment with Dr. D., also a male therapist. Dr. D., realizing that Agnes's chronic complaints were unconscious wishes, did not try to get Agnes to manipulate and alter Charlie's behavior; he knew she derived gratification and protection from living with a weak, passive man. Instead, he helped her explore her struggles and waited for her to experience her internal struggles with men in the transference with him.

A turning point in Agnes's therapy took place during her seventh month of treatment. In one session Agnes told Dr. D. that it was her birthday over the weekend. In anger she declared, "What did Charlie give me for my birthday? Some stinking perfume and some old flowers! Plus, he took me to a lousy restaurant and we had lousy food!"

When Dr. D. did not say anything about Agnes's complaints, after a minute of silence Agnes told Dr. D. she was quite sure that if she were married to Dr. D. he would have been more attentive to her needs. He would have given her a "fragrant" perfume and "nice" flowers and taken her to "an elegant and romantic restaurant" where they "would have a ball." When Dr. D. again listened attentively but did not comment, Agnes broke out into a rage. She told Dr. D. that he was "a rigid Freudian," "a pompous ass," and "didn't know a damned thing about women."

As Agnes could eventually see that her contempt for her husband was similar to her contempt for her therapist, she realized how she was punishing all men because of her frustrating relationships with her father and brother. To let a man be strong made her feel weak. Consequently, she tried to be strong and critical and keep her man weak.

The Extramarital Affair

A frequent marital problem brought to the therapist's office is the extramarital affair. What is frequently overlooked by many patients and therapists is that, when a person comes to a therapist with this problem, the patient unconsciously wants the equivalent of two spouses—one partner is insufficient.

If the clinician is not aware of the fact that the patient with two partners unconsciously derives gratification and protection from this arrangement, she is apt to try to influence the patient to give up the affair or give up his wife. This rarely works! The patient's internal struggle has to be addressed.

To understand a patient in an extramarital affair, it is necessary to get in tune with his specific unresolved maturational conflicts (Strean 1980). The man or woman in an extramarital affair is always a conflicted human being who has enormous difficulty sustaining an intimate relationship with one partner. Often he is very frightened of intense dependency wishes. Therefore, by having two mates, he deceives himself into feeling more autonomous. Or the patient may be one who is in an unresolved power struggle with the spouse; the affair gratifies his wish to rebel and undo the noose that binds him. And many patients unconsciously turn the spouse into a parental figure, which makes sex with the partner anxiety provoking. Therefore, somebody who does not remind him of home and mother is less upsetting to him.

In effect, the patient involved in an affair is still a child, and unless these aforementioned issues are addressed in the therapy the patient will not resolve his internal dilemmas. Many therapists are inclined to view their roles as a punitive or benevolent superego to the patient. I have observed many clinicians tell the patient that this behavior is "acting out" and "destructive" and he should cease and desist. On the other hand, I have also worked with clinicians who encourage the patient to have the affair under the guise of the therapist try-ing to be an accepting parental figure to the patient. Neither approach yields many therapeutic dividends.

As with other marital problems, the patient's unique transference reactions and specific resistances must be ad-dressed in the therapy—not merely the external behavior that the patient constantly discusses.

Ed, a married man in his early thirties, came to see Ms. F., a therapist in private practice, "in order to try to resolve" his affair. Married for five years, Ed found his wife to be bor-ing, asexual, and "had a noose" around him that was much like the noose his mother had around him when he was a young boy. In addition, Ed was frequently sexually impotent with his wife and justified his affair with his unmarried girl-friend because he was "always in great shape with her."

Ms. F. did not take any stand with Ed about his affair. She patiently and empathically listened to Ed's complaints about his wife, as well as his passionate declarations about his girlfriend. During the fourth month of treatment when Ed said he was thinking of leaving his wife and moving in with his girlfriend, Ed asked Ms. F. what she thought about the idea. In response, Ms. F. suggested, "Let's imagine to-gether what it would be like."

Although Ed was clearly ambivalent about leaving his wife, he tended to lean in the direction of leaving her, and in the sixth month of treatment went away with his girlfriend and lived together as husband and wife for a couple of weeks. Interestingly, as Ed's girlfriend enacted the role of a traditional wife and cooked for him and such, Ed became impotent with her!

Ms. F., with Ed agreeing, pointed out that in a close living situation with a woman, Ed became anxious and began to see his partner (regardless of who she was) as a mother figure. As Ed reflected more on this conflict, he increased his therapy with Ms. F. from twice to three times per week. By his ninth month of therapy Ed could clearly perceive that when he got very close to a woman and he made her a mother, sex felt like incest and he had to, albeit unconsciously, inhibit himself. This caused his impotence.

What was also particularly revealing as well as helpful to Ed was an exploration of his transference reactions to Ms. F. As he increased his sessions to three times a week and became more involved with Ms. F. emotionally, he soon found himself coming late to sessions and canceling several. When Ms. F. pointed out to him that he was avoiding her, he became indignant and told her that she was "a controlling bitch who was trying to tie a noose" around his neck. Eventually he could see that just as with his wife and girlfriend, when the relationship became close with Ms. F. Ed turned her into an incestuous mother and had to avoid her. He also could realize that his anger toward these women was his way of denying his feelings of weakness and smallness next to them.

As Ed was helped to face his internalized and lifelong struggles with his mother (and therefore with all women), he could feel more comfortable with his wife and gave up his affair.

Sexual Problems

Many married as well as unmarried men and women bring their sexual problems to the therapist's office. Although they don't enjoy their sexual problems, almost all of them fail to realize that they are unconsciously writing their own scripts and are frightened to have sexual pleasure. What many patients and therapists tend to overlook as they work on the patient's sexual problems is that how a person functions and relates sexually is based on the story of his life, his fantasies, introjects, and other internalized variables. That is why instructions and information on how to have better sex have had limited results (Strean 1983).

In order for a patient to resolve his sexual inhibitions, he has to find out why he wants them in the first place. Few patients are consciously aware that by inhibiting themselves sexually, they are trying to avoid their sexual partner. As we have already noted, it is easy to turn the partner into a parental figure and then feel like a weak, guilty child next to the partner. Sometimes a sexual problem reflects envy and competition with the partner and often the patient can be in competition with a real or imagined rival. All of these issues weaken sexual pleasure.

Unless the clinician can acquaint the patient with how he is distorting the sexual experience because he is not being sensitive to the child in himself, the patient's sexual problems will not be appreciably lessened. However, if the patient gets in touch with the child in himself, he can be a happier and more sexual adult.

Grace, a 24-year-old recently married woman, came into treatment with Dr. H., a male therapist, because she was sexually unresponsive to her husband of a few months. Having sex was so troublesome for Grace that she couldn't permit her husband to penetrate her. She would become tense and be in so much pain that even casual foreplay could not take place.

In her therapy with Dr. H., Grace was verbally inhibited and there were many silent lapses in her sessions. When Dr. H. pointed out to her that apparently she felt the same kind of discomfort with him as she did with her husband, Grace denied this. Her repudiating Dr. H.'s interventions was similar to her repudiating the idea of her husband penetrating her.

As Dr. H. patiently showed Grace that she was carrying on a war with him, with her husband, and perhaps other men as well, Grace unleashed a great deal of hostility toward him, telling him he was "insensitive and hostile." This was followed by much berating of her husband in and out of her therapy sessions. Eventually Grace could get to the real source of her sexual difficulties—a relationship with a father who was very tyrannical, controlling, and hostile.

As Grace could see how she was continuing a futile battle with her father in her marriage, her sex life improved by leaps and bounds.

PARENT–CHILD CONFLICTS

One of the least understood axioms of psychotherapeutic practice is that parents are constantly reliving their emotional and interpersonal pasts through their children. Many practitioners fail to realize that when a parent seeks a therapist's help in coping with his child, the presenting problem of the child's is really a description of the parents as well. For example, when parents aver, "My child does not respond to limits," they are subtly acknowledging that they become anxious when they try to limit their children and that they are conflicted about it. Similarly, when a parent says, "My child is not ready to hear about sex," the parent is revealing that he is not ready to talk about sex.

As Yonata Feldman (1958) stated close to forty years ago, "Whatever a parent's reason for coming for help with his child's difficulties, sooner or later we become aware that the parent, too, is emotionally disturbed now or was emotionally disturbed as a child, and that his or her difficulties are very similar to the child's. The more we study the parent, the more we see the similarity of the disturbance" (p. 23).

Clinicians have noted that parents of acting-out children offer them subtle rewards for their behavior and help the children behave as they behaved or would have liked to behave (Love and Mayer 1970). They have also observed that parents of neurotically inhibited children characteristically prevent assertive behavior in their children because such behavior induces anxiety in the parents. They withdraw friendliness and other forms of positive recognition except on those occasions when the child inhibits himself or submits to parental dictates (Sternbach 1947). The child becomes unwilling to relinquish neurotic or acting-out pleasures because he is so frequently the recipient of love premiums when he demonstrates his sensitivity and acquiescence to parental desires.

Just as a husband's complaints of his wife say as much about him as they do about the wife, what a parent cannot tolerate in his child is also what he cannot tolerate in himself. This is why advising a parent on how to behave with his child has limited results. The parent, in order to cope better with the child, needs help with his own unresolved maturational problems.

Ian J., aged 11, was referred to a mental health clinic because his reading level was much below his capacity. Despite his poor reading performance, most of his ego functions such as judgment, reality testing, and relations with people were quite mature. Further, his history showed that essentially nothing appeared eventful or traumatic.

As reports from Mrs. J. were reviewed and as her interaction with Ian was observed, it became clear that almost every time Ian asserted himself, Mrs. J. would squelch his spontaneity and finish his sentences for him. Ian, in effect, was obeying an unconscious mandate from his mother, which was: "Don't assert yourself! Don't be too individuated! I am your mouthpiece, and in many ways I am your eyes and ears too!"

When Ian began therapy, Mrs. J. announced that she had divorced Ian's father after he began psychotherapy. She also felt very antagonistic toward Ian's therapist, and constantly told Ian that he was not being helped. When Ian actually did improve his reading, Mrs. J. made her most determined effort to stop Ian's therapy.

Although Ian was helped in therapy to be more comfortable with his aggression, Mrs. J. needed to look at what frightened her about having an assertive, independent son. It was not until she got in tune with her enormous competition with and hatred toward men that Ian was able to read and assert himself in other ways.

The case of Ian J. helps us understand that a child cannot overcome his maturational conflicts until the parent does the same with his own struggles. Therefore, when a parent is having difficulty with a child, he needs help in seeing what is threatening to him about the child and/or what gratifications he unconsciously derives from the child's maladaptive functioning.

Those of us who have worked with parents who have conflicted relationships with their children repeatedly note that the parents unconsciously reward their children for maintaining a regressed position that they, the parents, enjoy vicariously. A parent may unconsciously prohibit a child's further psychosocial growth, not out of malice, but because such growth would activate the adult's unbearable anxiety. Unprepared for emotionally healthy living because he himself was improperly nurtured, the parent maintains a relationship with his child that is dynamically similar to the one he experienced in his own childhood.

THE UNATTACHED PATIENT

The caseloads of therapists are populated by many unattached men and women. Sometimes unattached men or women appear at the therapist's office experiencing dejection, desperation, and depression. Occasionally they are abusing drugs or alcohol. Not infrequently they boast that the men or women they befriend are passionately in love with them but they themselves can never get "turned on." Some of them are divorced, many have never been married, not a few flee from one relationship after another. Yet they share one thing—a deep yearning for a partner and a conviction that the single life is not completely fulfilling (Strean 1995a).

Just as married individuals who have conflicted marriages frequently ascribe the source of their difficulties to the mate and/or the marital institution, unattached men and women do something similar. They often say they are not meeting the right people, but don't know why. A very frequent complaint of theirs is that all the mature and desirable partners have been taken. Not infrequently, practitioners hear erudite presentations from their single patients that offer sociological proof that the status of the single person is largely engineered by a dysfunctional society.

What is crucial in helping unattached patients to move toward a sustained, intimate relationship is to show them how and why an unattached position offers them both gratification and protection. Many therapists overlook this truism and most unattached patients find it difficult to accept that they are unconsciously creating their own misery.

Advising single people to go to parties and other social events, prompting them on how to behave on dates, and telling them to take out personal ads have limited results. These patients need to see how and why they are driving potential partners away; their competition, hostility, sexual fears, and low self-esteem need intensive examination. Frequently, these patients need to see how they are recapitulating unsatisfying and destructive relationships from the past, often turning potential partners into ambivalent parental and/or sibling figures.

One of the common sources of difficulty for the unattached patient is that he makes the potential partner into a forbidden but very much desired parental figure. Usually, the best way to resolve this internal dilemma is by examining how it manifests itself in the transference relationship with the therapist.

Kathleen was a single woman in her mid-forties who had many years of unsuccessful therapy with a variety of therapists. Although all of her therapists were well-meaning and supported her many efforts in locating men, they all failed to show her how she was writing her own self-destructive script.

In her seventh attempt at therapy with Dr. L., a male, Kathleen was helped to see how she kept men at a distance by Dr. L.'s focusing sharply and extensively with her on her transference reactions to him. For example, Dr. L. noted that Kathleen would avoid looking at him in sessions. Most of his interpretations were politely rejected, and when she had negative reactions to Dr. L. she would cancel appointments and gossip about him with others.

As Dr. L. constantly showed Kathleen how she was distancing herself from him and subtly but frequently attacking him, Kathleen began to gain some conviction about how she was pushing men away. Slowly, she could see how she was recapitulating a sadomasochistic relationship with her father, and emulating her mother, who was very contemptuous of her father.

Working on her negative transference reactions eventually helped Kathleen to act out less hostility toward men, so that after two years of twice-a-week therapy she did get married and sustained a positive relationship with her husband.

Psychotherapy for unattached men and women with a focus on their psychosexual development, and with adherence to dynamic concepts in the therapy such as transference, countertransference, resistance, and counterresistance can help many lonely, angry individuals become able to enjoy a warm, intimate, and gratifying relationship with a loving partner.

WORK PROBLEMS

When patients describe their work problems, they often appear as if they are being exploited and are the victims of an insensitive boss and/or an oppressive work environment. Although their descriptions of their work environment and the individuals in it are often realistic, this is only half the story. People who have difficulties on the job are often acting out resentments toward parents and siblings, have difficulties with success, and are oppressed by punitive superegos, as well as by a host of other internal variables.

It is quite easy for therapists to advise patients to leave their jobs so that their lives can be better. However, as experienced clinicians have learned, job switching or behavioral changes on the job cannot appreciably alter a patient's work satisfaction until he knows himself better.

Wrecked by Success

A number of men and women with work problems who end up in therapists' offices have not been able to tolerate success. Without knowing why, they become depressed and dejected after a promotion and/or a big raise in salary. They are not aware that their success is experienced as a hostile, destructive act, and this is what they need to learn about in their therapy.

> Morris, a married man in his early fifties, had made the rounds. He saw career counselors, headhunters, psychotherapists, and other experts. Throughout his work life he went from job to job as a business administrator, and after an initial feeling of enthusiasm and optimism he lost interest in his work and often became depressed. His behavior with counselors and therapists paralleled his unsuccessful adaptation on jobs.
>
> Although Morris took all kinds of vocational tests and made many job changes to better suit his interests and skills, he still continued to be unhappy and left many jobs. Advice on how to relate better to peers and superiors did not appreciably alter his job dissatisfactions. Changes of residence to live nearer or further away from the jobs also did not help him.
>
> It was not until Morris went into psychotherapy with Ms. N. that his job problems diminished so that he could

enjoy his work much more. Ms. N. noted that Morris's enthusiasm on the job always lessened right after he received either a promotion or a raise in salary. As she explored this observation with Morris, they were able to learn that Morris felt very uncomfortable whenever he was in a superior position to his peers. It was even worse when he was considered part of management.

As Ms. N. and Morris studied his discomfort with success, it became clear that Morris experienced his elevations in status and salary as if he were "Joseph in the Bible." Consequently, he felt as if he was being contemptuous of his two brothers. Rather than "be thrown out of the house" by his brothers and feel enormously humiliated, Morris left the job first.

Seeing how he was constantly reliving his competition with his brothers, and getting in better touch with his hostility and need for punishment helped Morris learn to enjoy his job situation and stay with it.

When patients who have work problems want to quit therapy, often it is because they have not been sensitized to why leaving the scene is more comfortable than facing what is causing the anxiety. Although guilt about surpassing siblings and parents is a common cause, other conflicts can also cause job dissatisfaction.

Wishes Come True

Why do many men, women, and children want to believe that what they honestly worked hard for is the equivalent of stolen goods? One of the most apparent characteristics of children is they want what they want when they want it. They have very limited tolerance for frustration; to control impulses is very difficult for them. Consequently, children aggressively want to take what they see in sight that seems valuable and/or enjoyable. They "play house" and want to pretend they are adults. They "play doctor" and want to satisfy their sexual curiosity immediately. They "play school" and become the taskmaster rather than the student.

Because Morris in the case just discussed, like all of us, had powerful wishes to get as much and as fast as he possibly could, he had daydreams of beating up his brothers, taking all their strength away from them, and making their strengths his own possessions. When he was a young boy, he also had fantasies of being bigger than his tall father and making more money than he thought his father had earned.

In effect, when Morris became an executive, he began to believe that all of his "nasty dreams" had come true. For Morris to be a senior member in the workplace meant he had beaten up his brothers, stolen his father's business and income, made his mother consider him her favorite, and scoffed at all of his inferior companions in his old neighborhood.

Delusions of Power

Because we are small, vulnerable, and needy when we are young children, we aspire to be a Superman, a Batman, a Wonder Woman, or even God. These wishes do not leave us when we are adults because the nature of the human condition continues to be a vulnerable and imperfect one. Consequently, like Morris, many people can easily distort a realistic and laudable accomplishment and think they've become excessively powerful. Having wiped out others and thinking they have acquired so much, they feel very guilty toward those they think they have weakened. Thus, they punish themselves because they falsely believe they have weakened others.

Many of our patients would not feel like failures or provoke failure in their work if they could permit themselves to view their achievements more realistically. I recall a patient of mine, Peter, who was a salesman. Every time he made a major sale he went into a depression. When I explored with him how he felt immediately after a successful sale, he said, "I feel that I made a killing." Many salesmen and people in other pursuits want to believe they've killed one or more individuals when they are successful. Then they feel so guilty about their murderous wishes that they symbolically kill themselves to atone for their sins.

Very often I have to tell depressed, suicidal individuals who are suffering from much guilt that they are not as powerful as they think they are. Just because they have wished to destroy parents, siblings, and others does not mean they have succeeded in doing so. When I reminded Peter a few times that he might have wished to knock off his parents and siblings but was not as successful a killer as he thought, his guilt lessened and he could begin to enjoy his real abilities and talents without suffering so much.

In order to enjoy work and cope with its inevitable frustrations, one thing that helps our patients is accepting the fact that everybody on the job, including the patient himself, is in many ways still a child. Although they are in their twenties, thirties, forties, or older, there is a child in all of our patients wanting to be the most loved and appreciated individual in the job setting. They want constant praise and abhor criticism. They wish to yell or cry when things do not go their way. When they are tired they want to go to sleep or go home.

Once our patients recognize and accept the child in themselves, their competitive fantasies, hostile reactions, desires for revenge, and chronic ambitiousness do not overwhelm them as much. They realize they exist in everyone and they are not unique. Then they can begin to see themselves and their colleagues more realistically and the workplace does not appear as ominous. When my patient, Peter, could become in better tune with the little boy in himself who wanted to replace his father as head of the family and annihilate his siblings, his similar feelings toward his superiors and colleagues became less frightening and easier to monitor. As he was less critical of himself for being a hungry, ambitious, competitive child, he became more of a responsible adult.

The major issue for the practitioner to keep in mind when treating patients with work problems is that the workplace itself is not the only cause of the patient's plight. His history, fantasies, and conflicts must be addressed and given priority.

GENDER, RACIAL, AND RELIGIOUS DIFFICULTIES

One of the accomplishments of our contemporary society is having somewhat diminished sexism, racism, and religious intolerance. Frequently, mental health practitioners have been in the forefront in sensitizing others to the fact that we are all more human than otherwise (Sullivan 1953). As a result, all of us, patients, therapists, and others, have more freedom in declaring our indignation when we or others are discriminated against.

A very challenging patient is the one who uses his minority status as a defense to ward off other personal vulnerabilities. Even very talented and experienced clinicians have felt very frustrated with the patient who ascribes his difficulties to his race, religion, or gender. The reason this patient is frustrating is that many of his complaints are realistic and legitimate, but it is also clear that he is using them as a resistance. To suggest to the patient that he is overreacting is an invitation to have him quit therapy. However, if the patient's complaints are supported, he will become suspicious of the therapist because he knows on some level that he is being less than candid with him. Therefore, he will probably want to move away from therapy.

I have found that the most expedient way to help the patient we are discussing is to address the patient's complaints the same way we have prescribed for the treatment of marital complaints, parent–child problems, and other reality issues that we have confronted in this chapter. What I am referring to is working with the patient's transference reactions and showing him that he feels discriminated against by the therapist in the same way he feels oppressed by others. If the practitioner keeps in mind that chronic complaints are unconscious wishes, then she will be able to help the patient see how he arranges to feel oppressed. Most of the time he realizes, eventually, that he is using the opportunity to discharge some of his intense hostility by feeling persecuted.

> Rachel, in her thirties, came into therapy with Ms. S., a practitioner in private practice, for help with many problems. She was very unhappy on her job as a social worker, felt very angry at the men she dated, and resented the woman with whom she shared an apartment.
>
> As Rachel discussed her problems with Ms. S., she ascribed most of them to the fact that she was an orthodox Jewish woman and was scapegoated because of her religion and her gender. Ms. S. did not comment very much but patiently listened to Rachel as she vented her anger and felt very sorry for herself.
>
> During Rachel's sixth month in treatment, she berated Ms. S. for not "supporting, affirming, and reinforcing" her and threatened to quit therapy. When Ms. S. asked Rachel why she thought she was so withholding, rather spontaneously Rachel blurted out, "Because I am an orthodox Jewish woman." Then recalling that Ms. S. herself was also an orthodox Jewish woman, Rachel had to question her preoccupation with her gender and religious affiliation.
>
> As Rachel explored her feelings, she acknowledged that all her life she wanted to "tell off" her parents and others for "making" her feel "unwanted" as compared to how her brothers were treated. Frightened of her hostility toward her parents and parental figures, she displaced this problem onto her gender and religion.

BODY IMAGE PROBLEMS

A very common presenting problem brought in by many patients is a preoccupation with their poor appearance and weak body image. Frequently there is little basis in reality for the patient's negative self-image but he nonetheless clings to his excessive preoccupation with his baldness, thinness, or small penis. This patient tries all kinds of cosmetic and other remedies and pays lots of money to try to improve himself.

The patient's efforts to improve himself usually get him nowhere, as do the efforts of the therapist to support, praise, or decondition him. Sometimes the therapist can get taken in by the patient's preoccupations and offer suggestions as to how he can compensate for his problems of small size and other seeming irregularities. This, of course, compounds the patient's shame and low self-esteem because all it does is call attention to a displaced problem.

Experienced clinicians have learned the hard way that patients who call attention to their body image problems are avoiding issues and not confronting them. The man who talks about his small penis unconsciously wants to be a little boy and is frightened to compete with men. The same can be said of the woman who contends her breasts are too small—she is afraid to be part of the adult women's world.

Tom, in his mid-twenties, was in treatment because he had difficulties dating women. He was very self-conscious, shy, and tongue-tied with women, blaming most of it on his short height, which was about five feet, six inches.

As Tom discussed his problems with Dr. U., a male therapist, treatment yielded no results. Dr. U. tried to reassure Tom that he was tall enough but Tom was adamant, saying Dr. U. was too reassuring. When Dr. U. tried to get Tom to "accept" his limitations because there was "nothing" he could do about them, Tom fought this argument as well. When he left treatment, he told Dr. U. that he felt misunderstood and unsupported.

In his treatment with Ms. V., Tom was helped to talk about his history and his family relationships. Eventually he could face his strong and erotic relationship with his "seductive" mother. As Tom talked about his forbidden, sexual desires toward his mother, he could see why he needed to feel castrated and small.

Tom was particularly helped by facing some of his fantasies toward Ms. V. As Ms. V. did not censure him for his sexual desires toward her, he could feel a lot freer with other women.

As we have stated throughout this chapter, patients (and frequently therapists as well) have a penchant to view the patient as a victim of circumstance. As long as the patient holds on to this view, his psychosocial functioning will not be enhanced; rather, he will tend to stay in a regressed position and not mature.

In order to resolve situational difficulties, patients need to focus on their internal difficulties. Manipulation of the patient's environment, advice, and other attempts to modify reality have very limited results. Rather, when we concentrate on the patient's transference reactions and resistances, and our countertransference responses and counterresistances, the patient's possibilities of mastering his situational problems are immeasurably increased.

CHAPTER SIX

How Subtle Resistances of the Patient Are Reinforced by the Therapist: A Major Factor in Patient Dropout

nless one has practiced psychotherapy for several years and/or has been a patient in psychotherapy for some time, it can appear baffling to any logical person that men, women, and children who seek therapeutic help and make many sacrifices to stay in it want to fight it as much as they do. Yet, as sure as night follows day, patients always put up barriers to the therapeutic relationship in the same self-destructive ways that they cope with their spouses, colleagues, children, bosses, and others.

What can be intriguing yet frustrating to practitioners is to note repeatedly that what the patient in the first interview says she wants to correct is rarely addressed in the therapy for a long time. As I reflect on my current practice, virtually every patient is recapitulating in her interactions with me what she stated at intake consistently bothered her and for which she wanted my help. The woman who said she found herself consistently rejecting men and wanted to stop doing that scolds me constantly about my many limitations and imperfections. The man who told me in our first interview that he hates himself for always being "a yes man" to everybody around him is extremely deferential toward me and compulsively complies with everything he thinks I want from him. The student who passive-aggressively arranges to fail in school never fails to be late for his sessions with me and occasionally forgets about them. The lady who sought my help because she was getting uncomfortable with her sexual promiscuity is constantly trying to seduce me, while the gentleman who wanted to overcome his extreme obesity frequently enters my office eating an ice cream cone.

While most of the resistive behaviors I have just noted are what Glover (1955) would label as "crass," most patients deal with the dangers they experience in the therapeutic situation with an array of more subtle resistances. They manage to get caught in traffic snarls and are late for their sessions from time to time. Or they repeatedly "don't get" what the therapist is trying to explain. Occasionally they can't remember their recent dreams or fantasies and "forget" about mentioning to the therapist important events in their current or past life. Some patients find themselves discussing their discomforts with and resentments toward the therapist and the therapeutic situation with colleagues and friends, but avoid confronting the therapist with this same material.

Inasmuch as all resistive behaviors, such as lateness, absences, gossiping about the therapist, psychosomatic reactions, failing to grasp interpretations and/or frequently disagreeing with them, are unconscious attempts to lessen the impact of the therapist's influence, therapists are going to react to their patients' efforts to undermine them in their own characteristic ways. The therapist who wants to avoid the patient's expressions of the negative transference will tend to avoid exploring the meaning of the patient's lateness, absences, nonpayment of fees, and so forth. On the other hand, the practitioner who feels attacked by the patient's resistive behavior might subtly attack the patient with sharp confrontations and penetrating interpretations.

Just as patients can be excessively compliant, so can therapists. All the resistances we see in our patients can emerge as counterresistances of therapists (Strean 1993). Therapists are not exempt from being late for sessions, not hearing important utterances from their patients, or getting ill in the sessions.

Just as the responsible and competent practitioner wants to sensitize himself to the dangers that patients try to protect themselves from when they resist, he should also become aware of the dangers that he is attempting to avoid when he utilizes his habitual counterresistances. Is the practitioner afraid of being abandoned by the patient and therefore is too ingratiating? Is he angry because of the absence of love and admiration coming from the patient and therefore finds himself arriving late for interviews? Is he competitive and envious of the patient and therefore is constantly involved in power struggles with her? Perhaps he is afraid of his own sexual or aggressive fantasies toward the patient and therefore is too quiet and inhibited in the sessions.

One of the major reasons for patient dropout is that therapists, out of their own anxiety, fail to respond with understanding and empathy to their patients' lateness, absences, somatizations, or overcompliance. Instead, they may ignore the resistive behavior, subtly cooperate with it, or attack it without sufficiently monitoring their own hostility.

In this chapter my aim is to review and discuss several forms of subtle resistances that patients frequently exhibit and discuss how therapists respond to them. As in previous chapters, I will try to demonstrate how practitioners can be helpful or unhelpful in their attempts to help patients resolve their subtle expression of resistances.

In examining resistive behavior, whether it be the patient's or the therapist's, it is important to keep in mind that the form of behavior that the resistance takes has many different possible meanings. For example, a patient may be late for sessions because she wishes to defy the therapist. But she can also be late because she is afraid of her sexual fantasies and her desires for intimacy. Lateness may mask a desire to be punished (masochism) or to be noticed (exhibitionism). The same could be said about any other resistive behavior—it can have many different possible meanings. It is the mutual task of the therapist and patient to determine the meaning of the particular resistance.

LATENESS

Because therapists are busy people, they can welcome a patient being late so they can catch up with obligations such as phone calls and correspondence, or with pleasures like napping and reading. Occasionally the practitioner can find some of his patients to be irritating, trying, or boring and therefore might wish to ignore their lateness and enjoy being without them.

> Abe, a 40-year-old advertising executive, was in treatment because he was having a lot of difficulty on his job. He argued with colleagues and clients incessantly and felt irritable

when he planned his professional tasks. In addition, he found himself being very testy with his wife and children. In his initial consultation with his male therapist, Dr. B., Abe mentioned that he had always been in conflict with figures of authority during the entire course of his life. He wanted to alter this self-defeating pattern.

After a short honeymoon with Dr. B., during which time Abe felt a lot less tense, performed better on the job, and was less angry at home, he began to come late for his weekly therapy session. Dr. B. did not explore the lateness with Abe.

It was not until the eighth month of therapy when Abe made constant threats to end treatment that Dr. B. began to confront the fact that Abe had been constantly coming late for his sessions and that he, Dr. B., had ignored this resistance. As Dr. B. reviewed his work with Abe in supervision he realized how intimidated he felt next to Abe and was afraid that he would be attacked if he faced Abe with his lateness. Furthermore, Dr. B. became aware of the fact that he endowed Abe with all kinds of parental powers; consequently, to confront Abe with his lateness made Dr. B. feel like a little boy criticizing a powerful father. This seemed overwhelming to Dr. B. and he shuddered as he contemplated being the recipient of Abe's anger.

As Dr. B. could feel more willing to acknowledge some of his own hostility toward and fear of Abe, he became better prepared to discuss with Abe some of Abe's resentment and defiance that he felt toward the therapy and the therapist. As Abe could talk more freely of his resentments toward Dr. B. and the therapy, his lateness diminished and he began to function with much less hostility on the job and at home.

Just as lateness may be an expression of many different issues as we examine them in different patients, therapists vary among themselves in how they experience their patients' lateness. It is even possible for the same therapist to react differently to different patients' lateness and to find one patient's lateness meaning one thing to him at one stage of the therapy and something else at a later stage.

Very frequently therapists can experience the patient's lateness as a narcissistic injury. They feel hurt by the patient's behavior because they perceive it as an attack on themselves. Therapists, like all human beings, often cope with feeling attacked by subtly attacking the patient.

> Christina, a single woman in her early forties, was in treatment because she was becoming increasingly desperate about finding a mate. In her therapy with Ms. D., Christina was able to share with her how much she felt both intimidated and competitive with men. She was able to link this reaction to her relationship with her two brothers, who she felt "overpowered" her constantly during her childhood and adolescence.
>
> After several months of treatment during which Christina felt very much helped by Ms. D., who enjoyed Christina's "honesty and spontaneity," Christina's attitude drastically changed. Instead of appearing as a well-motivated patient, Christina became indifferent toward Ms. D. and the therapy. Her warmth and openness were replaced by coldness and tightness. When Ms. D. tried to explore Christina's change of attitude, Christina was reluctant to discuss it. Instead,

she began to arrive late for sessions and was unreceptive to any discussion of her behavior.

Ms. D. grew increasingly frustrated with Christina, and handled her annoyance by presenting Christina with sharp confrontations and hard-hitting interpretations. After Christina heard how defiant Ms. D. thought Christina was, and after being reminded many times by Ms. D. that she was reliving her relationship with her brothers in the transference, Christina reported that she had "had it" and quit treatment. She told Ms. D. that she felt disliked by her and needed to find "a more accepting therapist."

In evaluating the therapist's activity in the above case illustration, it is important to note that what Ms. D. told Christina about her lateness was correct. Christina was defying the therapist because she felt overpowered by a professional who reminded her of her brothers. What was missing from Ms. D. was an empathetic and understanding emotional response—not one that sounded judgmental and attacking.

After a therapist has been built up by a patient, it is not easy to take being torn down by her. One's narcissism is punctured and there is a strong temptation to attack the patient the way one has been attacked. Very frequently the patient "helps" the therapist counterattack because she unconsciously wants the therapist to "fight back" in order to feel that her own anger is justified.

What patients like Christina need is a great deal of patience from the practitioner. If the therapist can remind himself that the patient is feeling inferior to the therapist and that is why she wants to knock him down, he does not have to feel so narcissistically impoverished and also does not have to attack the patient to retaliate. Instead, he should try to show the patient that he understands how unpleasant it feels to be with him, how the therapeutic relationship is so reminiscent of irritating relationships in the patient's past, and how tempting it is to get into an argument with him.

It is only after a long period of testing the therapist to see if he will battle that the patient will think of diminishing her belligerent attitude. In order to modify her strong resistance, the patient has to have a therapist who handles his own punctured narcissism with understanding rather than with counterattacks, and with control rather than with impulsivity.

ABSENCES

While repeated lateness tends to express a passive-aggressive attitude toward the therapist and the therapeutic situation, continual absences tend to imply a fairly strong wish to reject both. In one way or another the patient, through her absences, is saying that she does not want to make her therapy or her therapist too important; other events have a higher priority.

There are many reasons why patients absent themselves from therapy sessions, and it is the job of the practitioner and the patient to try to figure out the reason or reasons. Patients can become frightened of their dependent wishes and worry that they will emerge as pathetic babies. They can also feel forced to submit to a parental figure and resent what seems like a rigid requirement. They can resent the therapist's power and authority. By being frequently absent from therapy sessions they may feel a little less dependent, less submissive, stronger, and more autonomous.

Frequent absences may be viewed as a form of acting out (Fenichel 1945), which means that the patient is acting on her feelings rather than expressing them verbally in the sessions and trying to understand what is causing her anxiety. Obviously, if the patient who acts out is frightened to face herself, telling her to stop being absent is only going to exacerbate her symptom. Many practitioners are being shortsighted when they tell a defiant patient to stop being defiant and to be cooperative instead. This usually leads to more defiance on the part of the patient.

I have found that one way to help the patient who is frequently absent begin to articulate her feelings rather than act them out is to have a fee policy that does not reward absences. When patients know they will be charged for a missed session if it can't be made up, they are more inclined to be present at sessions. This strengthens the possibility of their talking about their feelings simply because they are face-to-face with the therapist instead of being away from him.

As is true with all resistive behavior, the best way to resolve the issue of absences is if the therapist is more interested in understanding than judging them, more eager in sensitizing himself to the dangers and anxiety that the patient is feeling than in stopping absent behavior, and more ready to empathize than criticize. I have found that when the therapist tries to consider with himself and later with the patient how he might be contributing to the absent behavior, the patient is more willing to examine herself. Feeling less judged and less criticized, she is not as reluctant to reveal herself to the therapist.

Edgar, a young man in his early twenties, was in treatment with Mr. F. because he could not make up his mind about whether or not to be a practicing homosexual. Edgar "enjoyed" the first few months of therapy because to his surprise, Mr. F. did not try to influence him to be heterosexual, but attempted instead to help him discuss the issues and understand his ambivalence better.

After Edgar shared with the therapist that he was seriously thinking of having a homosexual affair, he began to miss therapy sessions. Although Mr. F. was quite sure that Edgar was finding it difficult to face him as he was moving toward the gay community, he wanted to make it as safe as he could for Edgar to talk about his absences in the sessions.

In one session Mr. F. said to Edgar, "I don't think I'm making it sufficiently comfortable for you to want to be here." Edgar strongly protested and told Mr. F. how compassionate and empathetic he thought Mr. F. was. Insightfully, he stated, "I think I want you to stop me from being a homosexual and since you won't, I resent you. But I know that my resentment is not rational so I ran from the whole damn thing."

When Mr. F. told Edgar that he could understand Edgar's resentment, given his wish to be curbed by Mr. F., Edgar was then able to bring out how much he viewed his homosexual wishes as "a punishment" that he wanted to give to his "seductive mother" and to his "sadistic and distant father."

As Edgar could voice his feelings toward Mr. F., particularly his resentment, he could eventually talk about his family relationships in his early life. Talking replaced action and Edgar's absences from sessions stopped.

Rarely mentioned in psychotherapeutic texts are the therapists' absences. Just as patients are frequently not conscious of their reasons for doing so when they are absent from sessions, therapists aren't always that aware either. Sometimes therapists can unconsciously arrange to be away from the office by going to professional conferences in order to avoid being with certain hostile patients. When the work becomes tedious and boring, therapists can take many vacations from their patients.

I have found that the best arrangement that the practitioner can make in order to reduce patients' absences as well as his own is for him to have a relatively fixed pattern of his vacations that patients know about well in advance. When the therapist sees that he is deviating from his pre-arranged vacation schedule with patients, he should begin to wonder about his own resistance to doing therapy at a particular time and to take seriously his patients' complaints about his absences.

Gwen, a single woman in her early thirties, was in treatment with Dr. H., a female psychiatrist. Gwen's major complaint at intake was that she was very afraid of intimate relationships with men, particularly sexually. When confronted with the possibility of sex, Gwen became very anxious and often felt like vomiting.

In the treatment situation Gwen did a lot of whining, complaining, and crying. She often appeared quite helpless and frequently asked Dr. H. for advice both in sessions and in between them. Around the seventh month of therapy Dr. H. began to take long weekend vacations that necessitated trying to rearrange Gwen's appointments. Gwen, a schoolteacher, could not easily get away from her classes and thus missed many therapy sessions.

Eventually Gwen began to accuse Dr. H. of disliking her, and suggested that she was trying to get rid of her. Dr. H. did not explore Gwen's associations but made interpretations, suggesting to Gwen that if she did not receive a lot of reassurance she felt rejected. Interestingly, Gwen agreed with Dr. H.'s interpretations and insightfully averred, "If I feel rejected so easily, why do you plan to be away from me so often? Well, now it's my turn. I'm leaving you!"

After a hiatus of a couple of months, Gwen went into treatment with Ms. I., a social worker in private practice. Although Ms. I. was also the object of Gwen's complaints, whining, and helplessness, and despite the fact that she had many fantasies of throwing Gwen out of treatment, she handled the transference–countertransference interaction much more judiciously than Dr. H. had done. First, Ms. I. had a relatively fixed vacation schedule that did not easily permit her or her patients to take off without thoroughly considering the implications of the absences. Secondly, when Ms. I. found herself irritated with Gwen, she slowly studied it and realized that the irritation she felt was probably similar to the irritation felt by the men who rejected Gwen. Finally, Ms. I. became convinced that it would be helpful to Gwen if she could study with Ms. I. how she alienated others with her childlike behavior.

During one of Gwen's "masochistic orgies" (Fine 1982), Ms. I. asked her what she was feeling. After several moments of reflection, Gwen concluded that she felt like a lonely little girl. As Gwen elaborated more on this state of being, Ms. I. asked her how she thought Ms. I. felt. To Ms. I.'s surprise, Gwen said, "I'd like you to feel sorry for me and want to mother me, but I guess you probably feel irritated with my constant crying."

Eventually Gwen and Ms. I. were able to get to the aggression Gwen felt that dominated much of her infantile behavior. As Gwen could express more of it, she became more interesting to herself and to Ms. I. Soon Ms. I. could stop fantasizing the discontinuance of the treatment and after a while patient and therapist agreed to increase the frequency of their sessions from twice to three times a week.

Whether the patient or the therapist habitually is absent, this is a sign that at least one of the parties is considering ending the relationship. If the therapist, despite his negative feelings toward the patient, wishes to see the treatment continue, he has an obligation to initiate a dialogue with the patient to try to ascertain the major dynamics contributing to the absences.

ACTING OUT THE TRANSFERENCE

Whenever a patient of mine in her sessions is expressing a great deal of affect toward someone in her environment and is also discussing the person's behavior and attitudes, I usually begin to hypothesize that the person who is preoccupying the patient is a stand-in for me. One of the inevitable occurrences in psychotherapy is that the patient is frequently unable and/or unwilling to show the therapist her sexual and aggressive fantasies. However, because these fantasies are seeking discharge, they become displaced onto other individuals in the patient's immediate environment (Freud 1905).

I remember treating a young man who, prior to almost every session with me, would have sex with a woman. It took me a while before I could figure out that my patient was trying in this way to cope with his homosexual fantasies toward me. Unable to face his erotic feelings toward me, he chose an attractive woman instead. This way he could deny his feelings about me—they were discharged before our sessions—and he could enjoy himself rather than suffer the agony of facing his sexual fantasies toward me.

I also recall a woman whose marriage began to deteriorate as she continued her treatment with me. It also took me a while, as in the previous case, to realize that the frustrations she felt in her therapy were not coming out and she was displacing the anger she felt toward me onto her husband. I was enjoying being the object of her praise and admiration, and therefore resisted facing that she also hated me for not gratifying her sufficiently.

Often a boss, colleague, or relative is the recipient of the slings and arrows that the patient wants to direct toward the therapist but is afraid to. However, even when it dawns on the practitioner that an acting out of the transference is taking place, it is not an easy task to sell this notion to the patient. As I have constantly stressed throughout this text, unless the patient herself has some conviction about the material presented by the therapist, the most brilliant and insightful interpretation in the world can go in one ear and out the other (Fine 1968). However, if the therapist uses his "third ear" (Reik 1941), he can help the patient become better sensitized to her current transference fantasies.

I have learned that the most expedient way to help a patient get in touch with the transference fantasies that are being acted out toward someone in her environment is to say very little—almost nothing—about her interactions with that person. When the patient's involvement with the displaced object is not responded to by the therapist, sooner or later she will begin to face her discomfort with what is transpiring in the relationship. This is usually preceded by attempts of the patient to get the therapist to take a position on the acting-out behavior and of course this should be avoided as much as possible.

> Josh, a 45-year-old college professor, was in treatment with Dr. K., a psychologist. Josh sought treatment because he was very depressed, had several psychosomatic problems, was in a poor marriage, and was very disappointed about his lack of professional progress at his university.

After a prolonged honeymoon during which Josh's depression lifted and his other problems seemed to decline, Josh became very involved in disputes with the dean at his university. Although Dr. K. was quick to recognize that Josh was acting out his first treatment crisis by displacing his feelings onto the dean rather than directing them toward him, Dr. K. just listened and did not make any comments about Josh's interactions with the dean. Eventually Josh asked Dr. K. what he thought about his relationship with the dean. Rather than give him an answer, Dr. K. asked Josh, "What are you feeling right now that prompts your question?" Josh then got irritated with Dr. K. and told him that he was "an ungiving bastard, just like the dean."

Josh, who had to begin to face the fact that Dr. K. could not be an omnipotent parent, displaced his hostility toward his therapist onto his boss—a very common occurrence in therapy. By being quiet and reflective, Dr. K. could help Josh better face his transference reactions toward him.

Although the resolution of the acting out of the transference usually takes much longer than it did in the case above, the treatment principles involved in the case of Josh remain the same for all acting-out patients. First, the practitioner must become aware that he is really the object of the patient's libidinal and aggressive desires. Second, he should not support or criticize the patient's actions, but merely listen to the patient's associations empathetically. Third, when the patient attempts to get the therapist to take a stand on the patient's behavior, the therapist should not comply but instead try to help the patient see what she is feeling that prompts her desire for the therapist to say something. Usually, when these steps are taken, the patient begins to experience some of the feelings toward the practitioner that she is feeling toward the displaced object.

NOT LISTENING TO THE THERAPIST'S REMARKS

Another frequent phenomenon appearing in the exchange between patient and therapist is the failure of the patient to listen and grasp the therapist's remarks. Although therapists have devoted considerable attention to their own failures in not being attentive to or not digesting the patient's associations (for example, Fine 1982, Greenson 1967, Strean 1990), they have not given sufficient attention to a similar resistance in patients.

Patients usually show their reluctance to listening in a subtle manner. They change the subject of discourse, but usually not too abruptly. They may quibble about the meaning of a particular word, or they may apologize and say that something is over their heads. They may also say, "I don't mean to interrupt you but something else that's extremely important just occurred to me and I must tell you now!" Usually the issue that was the subject of discussion is not resurrected.

It is essential for practitioners to keep in mind that when the patient fails to grasp the therapist's remarks more than once or twice in a session, or does so repeatedly over many sessions, this is not just a matter of cognitive slippage or intellectual dysfunctioning. Rather, the patient is finding the issue that the therapist is talking about anxiety-provoking. In effect, something is creating a danger for the patient.

Inasmuch as the patient's not listening to the therapist's remarks implies that she is trying to ward off sexual or aggressive thoughts, fantasies, memories, or deeds that arouse discomfort for her, the therapist's repeating what the patient failed to comprehend will serve no useful purpose. Rather, a presentation the second time can compound the resistance and the patient can start to use other means of escape—such as absenting herself from sessions or leaving therapy entirely. We have to repeatedly remind ourselves that when the patient isn't listening, she is scared.

In order to help the patient feel safe with the material before her, the therapist must address the patient's discomfort. One way that can be helpful is to share with the patient that what the therapist has been talking about is not too palatable to her.

> Lucy, a single woman in her early forties, was in treatment because she "still had not landed a husband" and her "biological clock was running out." After a brief honeymoon with her male therapist, Dr. M., she began to skip sessions, come late to others, and maintain a distance from the therapist by hardly ever looking at him when they conversed. When Dr. M. confronted Lucy with her lateness, absences, and distancing maneuvers, she invariably ignored him. Although uncomfortable being treated in this way, Dr. M. went along with Lucy's lack of involvement with him.
>
> When the pattern of ignoring him continued, Dr. M. confronted Lucy more often and more sharply. This only

intensified Lucy's resistances and she missed more sessions and came even later to others. Dr. M. realized that he was not responding to Lucy's resistances appropriately and sought some guidance.

After help from a colleague, the next time that Dr. M. was ignored by Lucy, he said, "I think I'm making our work difficult for you. Sometimes I feel like a nudge." Lucy was able for the first time in a long time to "feel understood" by Dr. M. She declared that she resented his "intrusiveness" and "overeagerness" to have his ideas "penetrate" her.

After having the opportunity to vent some of her animosity, Lucy was able to face some of her fears about being sexually penetrated and other fears of intimacy.

As I have suggested several times throughout this text, there are countless reasons why patients avoid therapists (and why therapists avoid patients). Not listening and failing to grasp the therapist's remarks are distancing maneuvers that emanate from the patient's anxiety. It is the patient's anxiety that must be addressed—not her auditory or linguistic capacities.

PSYCHOSOMATIC RESPONSES

One of the more recent findings in both the biological and psychological sciences is that the mind and body are *always* functioning interdependently (Finell 1997). Feelings, thoughts, memories, and fantasies, when not verbalized, are often expressed by headaches, gastrointestinal troubles, cardiac problems, and other bodily disorders. By the same token, hormonal deficiencies, circulatory problems, respiratory ailments, and other somatic disorders can influence one's psychological well-being.

As psychotherapy moves into its middle and later phases, and emotions and defenses are constantly being stimulated and challenged, the patient's anxiety usually increases. Therefore, the possibility of the patient's body taking over the expression of her conflicts is stronger; bodily aches and pains may appear more frequently than they ever have occurred in the patient's life. This can be very frightening to many patients, who are in therapy to get better, not worse. Sometimes therapists who are unprepared for this get frightened, too.

I have learned over the years that when a patient begins to somaticize, she is bringing her body to my attention, much as a helpless baby who can't talk yearns for a mother to hold her and soothe her (McDougall 1989). If the therapist, in loco parentis, pays sufficient attention to the patient's bodily complaints, asks pertinent questions about them, and empathizes with the patient, this activity often has a salutary effect. The child in the adult patient feels comforted and does not need to work so hard to bring her primitive needs to the practitioner's attention.

In addition to the tender love and care that the psychosomatic patient needs, she also has to be helped to verbalize the feelings that are being held back by her bodily symptoms. Often the feelings are transference reactions that the patient is frightened to reveal. A headache on the way to a session (or in the session) may be a way of holding back anger and tears that the patient can't feel free to show the therapist.

Deep breathing and circulatory symptoms may be defending against dependency wishes and other yearnings toward the therapist (Strean 1996b). Gastrointestinal problems may mask desires to defecate on the therapist.

If the patient feels empathized with and sufficiently soothed, she may be able to talk about and eventually express the emotions that are being hidden when the practitioner asks, "What do you suppose you can't stomach (or is in your head, or that's breaking your heart, or leaving you breathless) that is too difficult to tell me?"

> Norbert, in his early fifties, was in treatment with Dr. P., a female psychologist. He had recently experienced a business failure and when he came to see Dr. P. he was unemployed and depressed. The first few months of treatment were "enjoyable" for Norbert because he could talk to "an attentive and empathetic listener and feel loved." His depression lifted and he began to consider other business opportunities.
>
> As Norbert began discussing these other business possibilities, he started to develop stomachaches on the way to the sessions, as well as during the sessions. Dr. P., an experienced practitioner and a motherly person, paid a great deal of attention to Norbert's bodily complaints, asking him to describe the symptoms in detail, to recall their onset, and to remember the times in his life he had experienced them. This kind of interest from Dr. P. had the effect of calming Norbert and inducing in him a feeling of warmth toward Dr. P.
>
> When Dr. P. observed that a good therapeutic alliance had been established, she asked Norbert, "What thoughts about me are hard to stomach and are also difficult to tell

me?" After some hesitancy on Norbert's part, followed by some reassurance from Dr. P. that she welcomed hearing all that was on Norbert's mind, particularly at this time when it could possibly reduce his somatic problems, Norbert was able to "tell all." He confided that he was scared to go back to work, that he enjoyed being unemployed in many ways, and he was worried that Dr. P. would think less of him if he didn't go back to work.

Dr. P. lauded Norbert for his courage and honesty and reassured him that her interest was in understanding him, not in getting him back to work. With this kind of benign attitude coming from Dr. P., Norbert could take his time in discussing his anxieties before returning to business.

One of the less obvious aspects of psychosomatic responses is that the patient is like a preverbal baby. The therapist, in order to help this patient eventually feel comfortable enough to talk, should pattern his activity and attitude as if he were a parent ministering to a preverbal baby. If the baby is soothed, comforted, and loved long enough and unambivalently, she will begin to feel like talking to the therapist about the emotional conflicts that bother her (Strean 1996b).

LATE PAYMENT OF FEES

One way that many patients express their resentment toward the therapist is through the late payment of fees. Some patients have all kinds of rationalizations for this resistance, such as "a poor cash flow," "less income," "more expenses," and so forth. Although these issues are real in many ways, when examined in detail by the therapist he usually finds that the patient does not want to make the therapy or the therapist a top priority in her life.

As I have investigated with patients what is causing their late payments, I have often learned that the money that was initially allotted for therapy is now being used for something else. If I ask the patient how come she would rather pay the money for clothes, vacations, or something other than therapy, the hostility that has been held back often comes to the surface and I hear, "You are not that important" or "Therapy is a luxury" or "You make enough" or "I thought you cared about my welfare; now you want me to worry about yours?" I have rarely found a patient in strong, positive therapeutic alliance holding back fees; this tells us that delinquent payments are usually a reflection of underlying hostility toward the practitioner.

Although some patients tell the therapist that they recognize they are late in paying the fee, others prefer to ignore what they are doing. Therapists can be described similarly; some don't let a moment go by without mentioning the delinquent payment to the patient while others may ignore it altogether.

Late payment of fees, like all resistances, cannot be ignored. However, constant nagging by the therapist usually makes the patient more reluctant to pay the fee, and nothing much gets resolved this way. I do think it is important to ask a patient who is overdue in her payments by a couple of weeks or more if she is having difficulty with finances. I also believe, as was just mentioned, that it is imperative to explore her rationalizations for not paying so that her latent hostility can emerge. Usually, when the hostility comes out, money is not the predominant issue that is bothering the patient but something in the therapist–patient interaction.

Roslyn, married, in her early forties, was being seen in a family agency for marriage counseling by Ms. S., a social worker. Although Roslyn paid her monthly fees promptly for the first few months of treatment, this began to change. First, Roslyn was late by a week, which Ms. S. ignored. But soon Roslyn developed a pattern of paying three or four weeks late. Ms. S. decided to investigate the issue when the problem was becoming frequent and chronic. Ms. S. asked Roslyn, "Are you having some difficulty with finances? I notice that it's not easy to pay me on time." Roslyn responded, "I have a lot of expenses—piano lessons, church fees, the kids need clothes." When Ms. S. said, "I guess you feel these activities should be paid before you pay me," Roslyn became very angry and told Ms. S. that she made Roslyn's relationship with her "too important" and she resented Ms. S.'s "preoccupation" with herself "enormously."

As Roslyn berated Ms. S. for her "narcissism," "self-importance," and "egocentrism," she did begin to pay her fees on time. Although it took a long time for Roslyn to see that she was in a power struggle with Ms. S. and that much of the "narcissism" that she ascribed to her was a projection of her own, the more she could do this, the less she needed to act out her hostility by the late payment of fees.

Occasionally, despite all of the therapist's efforts at trying to understand the patient's resistance, certain patients refuse to pay their fees. When I see that a payment is six weeks overdue, I tell the patient that we will have to stop the therapy. I have found this mobilizes most patients to figure out a way to pay their overdue fees and helps them to examine what is going on in our relationship. I have noted that when a therapist is frightened to take this kind of stance, the debt keeps increasing and may never get reconciled. This obviously is not helpful for the patient's psychological welfare, or the therapist's either.

EXCESSIVE PREOCCUPATION WITH THE PAST, PRESENT, OR A PARTICULAR ISSUE

When patients are preoccupied with a particular issue, or excessively concerned with the past or present, usually they are trying to avoid facing something else; the preoccupation serves as a defense. For example, I had a patient who spent a good part of every session dwelling on her husband's physical weaknesses. I learned after a while that it was anxiety-provoking for her to think of him as a symptom-free and healthy man. I remember working with a man who talked only about his past; this preoccupation helped him avoid facing frightening events in the present, such as his heart condition and unemployment. A woman who obsessively dwelled on events in the present did so to avoid facing an ambivalent, erotic relationship with her father that traumatized her early in life.

Many therapists who understandably react with boredom and irritation to the patient's obsessiveness can handle their countertransference reactions by bombarding the patient with interpretations. Not consciously realizing they are indirectly telling the patient to shut up, they become very surprised when the patient responds to their interventions with indignation and then makes threats to leave treatment. (It is truly amazing how perceptive and sensitive patients are to their therapist's moods and motives!)

Like all resistances, obsessive preoccupations are utilized to protect patients against danger and discomfort. That is why the practitioner must respect the patient's defensive means of coping and not challenge them prematurely or aggressively; otherwise he may not have any patient! Although most clinicians do not consciously want to lose their patients, aggressive and premature interpretations, when used frequently with a patient, are often an unconscious attempt by the therapist to get rid of her.

> Tom, a man in his early sixties, was in treatment for depression, a poor marital relationship, sexual difficulties, and dissatisfaction on the job. In his therapy with Dr. U., a male psychiatrist, Tom spent most of his time talking about the health foods he ate and little else. Dr. U. kept telling Tom that he was avoiding facing very pertinent problems in his life by talking almost exclusively about his diet. Although Tom tried to comply with Dr. U.'s admonitions, he found himself repeatedly returning to his discussion of food. But, the more Tom discussed his diet, the more Dr. U. made interpretations about Tom's wish to regress to orality, his fear of sexuality,

his reluctance to have intimate relationships, and other "neurotic adaptations." Eventually Tom left treatment.

Although Dr. U.'s interpretations were accurate, Tom sensed they were motivated by Dr. U.'s annoyance and boredom. Feeling unloved, he left treatment.

A few months later Tom went into therapy with Mr. V., a social worker in private practice. When Tom deluged Mr. V. with his food habits and concerns about a healthy diet, Mr. V. patiently and interestedly asked Tom about further details of his diet. He even started off a couple of sessions by asking Tom, "How was your lunch today?" or "What did you have for supper last night?"

As Tom felt genuinely accepted by Mr. V., he could slowly share his chronic and embarrassing problems with him. Feeling respected, he could reveal some of his vulnerabilities. What appeared dangerous was no longer so ominous to face once he knew the therapist was an ally and not an opponent.

As we learned from the above case illustration, one of the best ways to keep a patient in treatment is to respect her resistances. When the patient feels supported and understood, she begins to feel more positive toward the therapist. If the therapist is viewed positively by the patient, he is more inclined to want to relate empathetically and a working alliance grows.

THE EXIT LINE

Many patients enter a therapy hour with conscious thoughts, feelings, plans, or memories but are very ambivalent about revealing them to the therapist. Consequently, they hold on to these thoughts, feelings, and such, and as they are about to leave the therapist's office they say, "I won't be here for the next session," or "I'm planning to get married this weekend," or "My wife and I decided to get a divorce," or "I really do love you," or "I really do hate you," or "I'm dropping a session as of next week."

These "exit lines" (Gabbard 1996) are like a neurotic symptom. They show that the patient is eager to discharge a wish or a feeling, for example, "I love you," or "I'm getting divorced," but the wish or feeling has to be defended against because it is too anxiety-provoking to discuss in the session. Thus, the compromise is the exit line.

Often therapists are startled to hear exit lines because they emerge as surprises that seem out of the blue, and sometimes it is not easy for therapists to hide their powerful reactions. I have responded to exit lines with spontaneous expletives, "Wow!," "Ouch!," or "No kidding."

Very often after I have responded with a startled reaction, I have found myself saying to the patient, "We have to talk about this!" And I have learned that most patients, although a little reluctant, essentially welcome the idea of the therapist wanting to talk about the issue at the next session. Otherwise, they probably would not have offered the exit line in the first place.

> Wendy, in her mid-thirties, left her therapist's office saying to her male therapist, Dr. Y., "I'm going to attend your lecture next Tuesday at the Y." Startled, Dr. Y. said loudly and anxiously, "No kidding!" Both therapist and patient then

turned red and became silent. Gathering his composure, Dr. Y. said, "Let's talk about it, okay?" Wendy remarked, "I will if I can."

In the next session, when Wendy did not bring up her wish to attend Dr. Y.'s lecture, Dr. Y. asked her, "How would you feel if we talked about your coming to my lecture?" After some hesitant starts, Wendy was able to discuss her wish to attend her therapist's lecture and said that she was fast becoming one of his ardent fans. This led to "a confession" of many erotic feelings toward Dr. Y., which Wendy began to think would be better discussed than her going to the lecture.

The exit line is the patient's awkward attempt to ask the therapist's help with a difficult issue in her life, which is why it is usually helpful, if the patient does not bring it up in the next session, for the therapist to do so. If it is too difficult for the patient to pursue, the therapist can acknowledge this and tactfully ask what the dangers are. Most patients welcome this approach.

"I'M CURED. LET'S STOP. THANK YOU VERY MUCH."

Every seasoned practitioner has had the experience of being told without notice that his patient feels cured and would like to stop treatment. Sometimes the wish is to terminate that particular day; occasionally the desire is to stop treatment within a couple of weeks.

When the patient without warning pronounces the edict of termination, we can usually infer that she cannot face certain transference feelings and wants to escape them. However, if we tell a patient who is eager to quit treatment to stay, she often becomes more adamant and can leave abruptly. Therefore, I have found that when a patient tells me without notice that she's leaving treatment shortly, I try my best *not* to challenge her but to listen carefully to her thoughts and plans.

Most patients, when they are not opposed, do one of two things, or both. Without being challenged they are able to begin voicing some of their indecision about quitting. This then allows the therapist to suggest toward the end of the session, "I think you haven't fully made up your mind. Perhaps we can spend a session or two looking at this some more." The ambivalent patient usually welcomes this approach.

The second reaction to the therapist's neutrality is to pose many patients' very popular question, "What do you think of this idea?" This question usually affords the therapist the opportunity to say, "I don't mind telling you. But let's see what you're feeling that prompts your interest in my position on this." Patients then can come out with more ease with just what they are currently feeling.

Tony, a man in his early forties, had been in treatment with Ms. T., a psychologist in private practice. He had sought therapy because he found that he was very unsuccessful in sustaining relationships with women. After a few months of treatment he reported that, though he wasn't in a relationship with a woman, he felt confident that he could be in one and was ready to leave treatment in a few weeks.

Despite the fact that Ms. T. realized that Tony was doing with her what he consistently had done with other women—leaving them when he felt uncomfortable with his sexual feelings—she knew she could not tell him this. Rather, she listened carefully to his thoughts and plans, was noncommital about her own stance, and said at the end of the session, "Let's talk some more about your decision at your next session," which was in two or three days.

At the next session Tony did acknowledge that during the last two days he had been irritable and hadn't slept well. When Ms. T. asked him to what he attributed this, he had no answer. Ms. T. then asked him how he felt about their last session. At first Tony forgot what they had discussed but later did remember that he had "some thoughts about ending our contact." After a long silence, Tony asked Ms. T., "How do you feel about ending our contact?"

When Ms. T. told Tony that she had some opinions but thought it would be helpful if he could say what he felt right now, Tony said, "I guess I'd like to know you want me to stay here. But I'm not sure you do." Ms. T. told Tony, "I think what's happening between you and me happens in your life a great deal. You are feeling warmly toward me, as you are quite capable of feeling toward a lot of women, but you're not sure that's okay with me." Tony said, "If I tell you I like you, you might say goodbye so I say goodbye first."

When faced with the patient who prematurely announces that treatment is over or should be terminated soon, it is crucial, if the therapy is going to be sustained, that the therapist not try to talk the patient out of her position. Rather, if he listens attentively, responds neutrally but empathetically, the patient will have a better opportunity to voice her feelings and look at some of her conflicts. As we saw in the above vignette, many times a professed desire to quit treatment is really a disguised cry to be asked to stay.

Threats to quit treatment arouse strong countertransference responses, which is why understanding our countertransference reactions is a prerequisite for good therapy—the subject of our next chapter.

CHAPTER SEVEN

FURTHER THOUGHTS ON COUNTERTRANSFERENCE REACTIONS: HOW THEY CAN INFLUENCE THE PATIENT'S WISH TO STOP TREATMENT

As has been noted several times in previous chapters, in order to help patients successfully complete their treatment, therapists need to be aware and in command of how they feel when they are the objects of their patients' emotions. How does the practitioner feel when a patient declares his "passionate" and "sincere" love for her? What becomes aroused for her when she is the object of a symbiotic transference and the patient constantly proclaims, "I can't live without you!" On the other side of the emotional spectrum, what does the therapist feel when she is very much hated by the patient and is the recipient of his constant contempt? Finally, what is induced in the mental health professional when the patient dogmatically declares that the treatment is ineffective, that she is incompetent, and that he is going to quit at the end of the session?

Not only does the therapist have to be sensitive to how she reacts to the patient's expressions of various affects and diverse coping mechanisms but, to do effective treatment and maintain the patient's involvement in it, she should be aware of her own, personalized transferences. Is she making the patient her mother or father? Or is she experiencing him as a sibling? Or as a lover? Or as a child? Or perhaps as a combination of all these?

Current mental health practitioners now view the countertransference very differently from the way their predecessors did. The modern therapist alleges that no psychotherapeutic phenomenon can be comprehensively assessed unless the therapist's countertransference reactions are given a great deal of attention and understanding. Therefore, no study of premature termination of therapy would be complete without a serious consideration of the role countertransference reactions play in patient dropout.

Before we examine those countertransference reactions that play a significant role in the premature ending of therapy, a word on the changing position of countertransference in the psychotherapeutic landscape may be of interest and help to the modern mental health practitioner.

From Freud's (1910) original dictum that "the countertransference arises [in the therapist] as a result of the patient's influence on his unconscious feelings, and we are almost inclined to insist that he shall recognize this countertransference in himself and overcome it" (pp. 144–145), current practitioners tend to view countertransference as including "all of the emotional reactions at work" (Abend 1989, p. 374). Rather than an obstacle to be overcome, countertransference is now regarded by most dynamically oriented clinicians as "all those reactions of [the therapist] to the patient that may help or hinder treatment" (Slakter 1987, p. 3).

There is now a rather large psychotherapeutic literature on countertransference, and most authors acknowledge that it is as ever-present as transference and must be constantly studied by all practitioners, from the neophyte to the very experienced (Abend 1982, 1989, Barchilon 1958, Boesky

1990, Brenner 1985, Fine 1982, Jacobs 1986, Kernberg 1965, Reich 1951, Renik 1993, Sandler 1976, Strean 1995b). Virtually all authors agree that, like transference, countertransference can frequently be subtle but is always an important influence on therapeutic outcome. Further, most writers concur that examining countertransference is no less difficult for the most experienced clinician than it is for the beginner.

The increased examination and discussion of countertransference has helped most clinicians to recognize that the psychotherapeutic process is always an interactive one. Boesky (1990) stated the issue clearly when he averred, "I consider the 'purity' of a theoretic treatment, in which all of the resistances are created only by the patient, to be a fiction. If [the therapist] does not get emotionally involved sooner or later in a manner that he had not intended, [the therapy] will not proceed to a successful conclusion" (p. 573). Just as there can be no therapy without constant transference reactions and resistances on the part of the patient, most current practitioners would contend that no therapy proceeds without constant countertransference reactions and counter-resistances on the part of the therapist.

Another illuminating insight that has evolved from the study of countertransference in greater breadth and depth is the current view that it is a central component in the therapist's use of treatment procedures. How and when the therapist is silent, poses questions, confronts, clarifies, and interprets, or uses parameters is based on her countertransference at the time of the intervention. Jacobs (1986) has demonstrated that psychotherapeutic technique is almost always a "countertransference enactment," even when the technical procedure is considered to be a valid and acceptable therapeutic intervention.

Perhaps one of the most valuable contributions to the study of countertransference enactments has been made by Renik (1993). Recognizing that the clinician's individual psychology constantly determines her therapeutic posture, Renik has clearly demonstrated that "awareness of countertransference is always retrospective, preceded by countertransference enactment" (p. 556). Just as no patient who is in the middle of a transference reaction is constantly aware of his distortion and does not say, for example, "I am now making you my seductive mother," the same may be said of the therapist and her countertransference responses. It is only after the countertransference enactment that the therapist may become aware of her personal involvement.

Renik (1993), like many other authors (for example, Brenner 1985, Fine 1982, Jacobs 1986) has demonstrated that the therapist "cannot eliminate, or even diminish his or her subjectivity" (p. 562). We are always personally involved as we make professional assessments, clinical decisions, and therapeutic interventions.

In a recent book, *The Power of Countertransference*, Maroda (1994) has creatively expanded on how countertransference reactions can be utilized to enrich the therapeutic process. She has clearly demonstrated how the therapist's neutrality can be used as a place for the therapist to hide from the patient and that the disclosure of countertransference reactions at times can be valuable and effective in working with all patients. Agreeing with Racker (1968) that it is a distortion of truth to view therapy as an interaction between a healthy clinician and a sick patient, Maroda has documented that "many of our patients will be healthier in some respects than we are, and even our sickest patients will understand parts of ourselves better than we do and will be strong where we are weak" (p. 14).

In formulating treatment interventions, Maroda has suggested, "The critical guiding factor for the therapist is the patient. The patient will tell you everything that you need to know, if you will only listen to him and consult with him" (pp. 21–22).

Stressing again and again that we all need to acknowledge that there is no such thing as therapist "neutrality," Maroda demonstrates repeatedly that all therapists each have their own personal axes to grind as they undertake each treatment. "We are there because we want something that goes beyond earning a living and beyond a commitment to social service or intellectual inquiry. We seek to be healed ourselves and we heal our old afflicted caretakers as we heal our patients" (pp. 37–38).

In applying Maroda's views to the subject before us, premature termination, one particular application has served me and my colleagues very well. As Maroda puts it, "I cannot state too strongly how unworkable I think it is to try to break a therapeutic stalemate without consulting the patient and enlisting his help" (p. 52).

Inasmuch as many books can be and have been written on the subject of countertransference, in this chapter we will limit our discussion and focus exclusively on those countertransference reactions that seem to provoke patient dropout the most. While the list is not exhaustive, I am quite sure the reader will find himself or herself in most of the categories that we will present.

THE FEAR OF IDENTIFYING WITH THE PATIENT

In order to conduct a meaningful treatment process to its successful conclusion, the therapist must be able to identify with the patient and experience his emotional struggles as if they were her own. Furthermore, not only must the therapist be able to step into the patient's shoes and experience his wishes, fears, guilts, and coping mechanisms, but she must also be able to master all of this emotional baggage and understand it well. This, of course, is an ideal to which we all aspire, but no therapist is able to achieve it without experiencing periodic regressions, showing blind spots, losing empathetic stances, and being unable to maintain objectivity.

When the therapist is unable to identify with the patient and feel his pain, understand his distortions, and empathize with his vulnerabilities, she can then become critical of the patient or impatient with him, withdraw from him, or become overactive with advice and/or environmental manipulations. One clue that can be useful in determining when the therapist is failing to identify with the patient is when she notes that she is not spending most of her time listening to the patient and trying to understand. Instead she may be talking too much or may become excessively withdrawn with her mind not concentrating on what the patient is producing.

When the clinician is afraid of her own pathology and primitive affects, she tends to move away from the patient's pathology and primitive affects. I believe that clinicians erect strong defenses against identifying with their patients when their patients' emotional struggles stir up in them similar struggles that they do not want to face. Usually this is not a conscious process. The therapist becomes aware of it only in hindsight (Renik 1993) and usually after the patient has given her some notion that, as far as he is concerned, the therapy is not going well.

> Anthony, in his early twenties, sought therapy because he had been jilted by his girlfriend, whom he had been dating for close to two years. Feeling extremely depressed, Anthony was sleeping poorly and eating little, and was castigating himself for all the mistakes he believed he had made in his interactions with his girlfriend.
>
> Dr. B., Anthony's therapist, was at first very sympathetic with Anthony's plight. He told Anthony that the loss of his girlfriend's love was a severe blow and he could understand why Anthony was suffering so much. Anthony welcomed Dr. B.'s support and for a while felt better.
>
> After some mild improvement, Anthony returned to his depressed state and brought out a great deal of agony in his sessions. This time Dr. B. tried to reassure Anthony and told him that he was quite able to find another girlfriend, and could even do better the next time.

Dr. B.'s reassurance had a negative effect on Anthony. He felt, with some validity, that Dr. B. was trying "to talk me out of feeling crummy" instead of letting him "mourn for the good old days." After being admonished, Dr. B. began to become impatient and critical with Anthony and this attitude of Dr. B.'s seemed to intensify Anthony's depression. Soon after, Anthony left Dr. B. and went to see another therapist.

When Dr. B. reviewed his work with a senior colleague, he was able to recall being jilted by a young woman when he was around Anthony's age. Never able to mourn his loss, Dr. B. defended himself against the primitive affects that were aroused in him when he was rejected by his girlfriend. When Anthony shared his agony and grief with Dr. B., Dr. B. could not tolerate hearing it because it reminded him too much of his own. Not able to face himself, he could not help Anthony deal with his own mourning.

Another way of moving away from one's patient is by pigeonholing him into a diagnostic category such as "borderline" or "psychopath." I have noticed in my own work and in the work of colleagues that when a patient is given a diagnostic label, it is usually an attempt to create distance between oneself and the patient, and this is motivated by the therapist's resentment and helplessness. Rather than face our feeling of similarity to a patient who is disturbing us, we call him "a disturbed person" and give him a label to make him as different from us as we can. Sooner or later the therapist's contempt is perceived by the patient, who then starts to think of quitting treatment.

Another way of coping with our resistance to identifying with the patient is by trying to change the treatment modality. I have found that when the therapist wants to give up individual treatment and move, for example, to conjoint treatment or family therapy, she is frequently trying to get away from the patient. What is imperative for the therapist to do when she feels inclined to alter the therapeutic modality is to study how she is feeling toward the patient and try to become sensitive to the part of herself that feels a wish to reject the patient.

Very often when a therapist wants to change the therapeutic modality, she turns to another therapist who is a specialist in it, such as group therapy, marital counseling, family therapy, and so forth. What she is doing, in effect, is saying, "Go see somebody else. I can't be with you full time!"

Identifying with the patient is a necessity. When it breaks down, it sooner or later leads to the patient quitting.

COMPETITION AND ENVY OF THE PATIENT

In any intense relationship between two people, competition and envy are inevitable. Although therapists generally try to help patients recognize these feelings toward themselves, few of them write or talk about how much they would like to possess some of the qualities their patients are fortunate to have. Hirsch (1980) states:

> Our patients are often younger, smarter, in better health, better looking, have more potential, have more excitement in their lives, have better relationships with

their loved ones, have more money, and on and on. [Therapists] who are unable to acknowledge both the fact of such differences and the ensuing jealousy or competitiveness run the risk of acting unconsciously to stifle the patients. [p. 127]

It has been my impression that many therapists cannot tolerate the inevitable competition, envy, and other negative emotions that are induced in them by patients. This, in turn, inhibits their capacity to help their patients deal with hatred and other negative feelings.

Maroda (1994) asks:

Are we leaning toward accepting a sugar-coated version of humanity that ultimately depersonalizes both therapist and patient, and unknowingly stifles the most positive human expressions in the process? How successful can we be in helping our patients to accept themselves when they are hateful, or petty and mean, or selfish and niggardly, if we cannot accept these feelings in ourselves? [p. 91]

When the therapist is unable to acknowledge her own competition and envy, the patient usually exploits this vulnerability in the therapist and a therapeutic impasse is likely. This may be followed by a termination.

Cathy was a single woman in her thirties, in therapy with Dr. D., a woman just a little older than Cathy. Seeking treatment because she was unable to sustain meaningful relationships with men, Cathy initially found Dr. D.'s patient and quiet listening quite liberating. Feeling more self-confident, she began to date men with more regularity.

Gradually Cathy began to get involved with a well-known entrepreneur who treated her like a princess. As Cathy bragged about being wined and dined and the recipient of all kinds of gifts, Dr. D. told Cathy that she was behaving like a little girl with an idealized father. As these kinds of interpretations began to mount, Cathy began to become depressed and told Dr. D. that she thought that Dr. D. was against her relationship with her boyfriend.

After being told that she was paranoid and couldn't appreciate Dr. D.'s kindness, Cathy quit treatment.

What was avoided by Dr. D. in the above case illustration? Clearly it was her reluctance to face her competitiveness and envy as Cathy became more loved and more successful. Had Dr. D. been able to face herself, she might have been more comfortable in helping Cathy see how much she wanted her therapist to be an envious lady.

As we have suggested, envy and competition in the therapist are inevitable. It is acknowledging it ourselves that will help us be more effective therapists.

FEAR OF THE PATIENT'S AFFECTS

One of the most important responsibilities of the psychotherapist is to help the patient feel free to reveal a full range of human emotion. Perhaps the main reason that our patients have neurotic symptoms, like insomnia, sexual inhibitions, phobias, obsessions, and compulsions as well as maladaptive character traits and problematic interpersonal relationships, is because they are not comfortable releasing their emotions anywhere to anyone. Frightened of their dependency wishes, overwhelmed by their aggressive fantasies, embarrassed by their sexual fantasies, and burdened by all kinds of ambivalence, our patients turn these struggles into psychological disorders.

In order to help patients gain confidence, increase their self-esteem, and diminish their symptomatology, character problems, and interpersonal stress, the therapist has to constantly relate to the dangers in the patient's psyche that block him from sharing his feelings with her.

Very often a patient's inhibitions are reinforced by the therapist, who has as much or more anxiety than the patient about facing certain feelings. It is not uncommon for therapists and patients to collude with each other, albeit unconsciously, and mutually avoid talking about issues like homosexual fantasies, aggressive wishes, competition and envy, romance, wishes to be a child and parent, and other affects.

I have often found it helpful to periodically review each patient I am working with and ask myself questions such as these: What haven't we talked about lately? Are we too much in the present? Are we too much in the past? Is the transference clear? What emotions haven't been directed toward me? Which emotions haven't I been feeling toward the patient?

Very often when there is a therapeutic impasse, the therapist has been unconsciously blocking the patient from releasing certain affects because these affects activate anxiety in her.

Ernest, a married man in his early thirties, had been in treatment with Ms. F., a therapist in private practice, for close to a year. Ernest entered treatment because of much job dissatisfaction and considerable marital conflict.

For a number of months the therapy seemed to be going quite well. Ernest was able to bring out in his sessions quite a bit of anger toward his boss at the accounting firm where he worked and do the same later as he discussed his wife with Ms. F. Ernest's self-esteem improved and both his work and marriage began to be much more gratifying to him.

When Ms. F. brought the case to a senior colleague for consultation after about one year of treatment, she reported to the consultant that Ernest had been missing a number of sessions, had been coming late to several, and had been talking with limited affect in almost all of them. Although Ms. F. knew that something in the transference–countertransference relationship was not being addressed, she could not be sure just what was happening.

As Ms. F. reviewed her work with Ernest in several consultations, it eventually became clear that after Ernest began to feel better, with some trepidation he tried to get closer to Ms. F. What also became clear was that Ms. F. was frightened of Ernest's growing warmth toward her and unconsciously blocked his attempts to get emotionally closer to her. The form this took was Ernest's asking Ms. F. questions about her own life, such as whether she was married, had children, and how come she became a therapist.

Rather than exploring with Ernest what he was feeling when he wanted to know more about Ms. F.'s life, Ms. F. responded coldly and unempathetically with responses like,

"Why do you ask?" or "What do you think?" Ernest felt rebuffed and rejected, and withdrew from Ms. F.

As Ms. F. studied her countertransference reactions, she realized that she was frightened of Ernest's sexual and loving feelings toward her and was also unable to enjoy her own sexual and loving feelings toward him. Thus, she made sure to create a distance between herself and her patient.

Fortunately the treatment was able to continue because Ms. F. shared some of her countertransference problems with Ernest. She told him that when he had asked her about her personal life, she subtly pushed him away rather than help him talk about what he was feeling toward her. Interestingly, Ernest was able to say insightfully, "You were afraid that we would fall in love with each other, right?" Although red-faced, Ms. F. could acknowledge the truth of Ernest's perceptions. Sensing that she was more accepting of her own loving and sexual feelings, Ernest could begin to talk about his erotic, maternal transference toward her.

Very often what can break a treatment impasse is when the therapist acknowledges the truth about her own contribution to the stalemate. Usually the truth has a lot to do with the therapist's resistance to experiencing affects of her own that are being stirred up by the patient, such as occurred with Ernest and Ms. F. In this regard, Maroda's (1994) sentiments are both pertinent and helpful.

> My response to those who fear that disclosure of the countertransference, even when done conservatively and at the patient's behest, will lead necessarily to "wild analysis" and unseemly gratification of the therapist's

personal needs, is simply this: more damage is done when the therapist hides than when he or she is direct and honest. I believe that more harm is done to patients by well-meaning therapists who do not want to "burden" their patients than by honest, straightforward clinicians who admit to the realities of doing therapy. [p. 174]

THE THERAPIST'S NEED TO BE LOVED AND ADMIRED

It has been well documented that therapists are "wounded healers" (Sussman 1992). Having suffered a great deal, part of their motivation in becoming clinicians is to cure themselves. One means of reassuring themselves that they are being effective healers is to hear from their patients that they are being healed, and one means that many clinicians use to feel they are doing their jobs properly is to arrange to hear from their patients how helpful, brilliant, and lovable they are.

While all human beings want to be loved and admired and therapists are certainly no exception, if the clinician's desire for approbation and gratitude is not carefully monitored, the danger of patient dropout increases considerably. There are many good reasons for this. First, the vast majority of patients have experienced their parents and parental figures as narcissistic individuals who had to be catered to and indulged; if the therapist is experienced the same way, the patient's mistrustful attitude toward the world continues and he does not feel helped. Second, if the patient feels obliged to always love, admire, and be indebted to the therapist, his aggression will go underground and his assertive capacities will be dormant. This, too, makes him question the therapy. Third, one of the goals of psychotherapy is to help the patient learn to like himself more, so that he will have less need for reinforcement and reassurance from others. A therapist who needs to be loved and admired a great deal is a poor role model for his patients. Patients usually end up feeling contempt toward the therapist and eventually quit therapy.

The clinician's need to be loved and admired can take many forms and has many negative repercussions. If the patient doesn't improve rapidly, the therapist can either become depressed or subtly critical of the patient and this, of course, interferes with the patient's emotional spontaneity in the therapy. The therapist may need to have his interpretations and other interventions accepted by the patient without qualification and this pressure grossly inhibits the patient's freedom to say what he feels and thinks. Other ways that the therapist can try to ingratiate himself are by heaping advice on the patient, encouraging dependency by extending therapeutic hours, and/or suggesting phone contacts between sessions. A fairly popular form of ingratiation by clinicians is keeping fees low and having too liberal a cancellation policy. All these examples of the therapist's childish narcissism (Finell 1985) can eventually lead to premature termination of the treatment. Finell points out that the therapeutic situation

> offers much gratification for [therapists] with intense
> needs to be loved, idealized, and to feel a sense of

power and control over others. [Therapists] with such dynamics will tend to promote idealization, power, and control by taking a dominant position in relation to the [patient] who is essentially submissive and masochistic in these dynamics. In these circumstances, [therapist] and patient collude and form a misalliance in the sense described by Langs (1975). The narcissistic character structure of both is protected, and both receive a great deal of gratification that leaves the basic pathology untouched. [p. 436]

Many patients who leave treatment prematurely have unconsciously sensed the therapist's childish narcissism and have realized that she is incapable of treating him competently (Maroda 1994).

Gladys, in her early twenties, was in treatment with Ms. H., a therapist in private practice. Gladys sought treatment because she was frequently depressed, felt too dependent on her parents, and was unsuccessful in sustaining relationships with men.

During the first few months of treatment, Ms. H. focused on Gladys's latent resentment toward her parents. This tended to diminish Gladys's depression and increased her self-confidence. As a result, Gladys felt very positively toward Ms. H. and repeatedly told her what an outstanding therapist and superb woman she was. Ms. H. enjoyed hearing Gladys's laudatory comments, expressed her gratitude frequently, and told Gladys that she was an excellent patient.

The love-and-be-loved relationship between therapist and patient shifted dramatically shortly after Gladys was told by

Ms. H. that she would be going on a month's vacation. Instead of her practice of coming to her sessions on time, Gladys began to arrive fifteen to twenty minutes late, and instead of being emotionally spontaneous, Gladys appeared lethargic and uninterested in the interviews. When Ms. H. pointed out these shifts in Gladys's attitude and behavior to her, Gladys told Ms. H. that she had changed her mind about her. Gladys said, "I used to think you were kind, considerate, and brilliant. Now I think you are selfish and stupid." Ms. H. took Gladys's statements very personally. At first, she responded with stiffness in her body and coldness in her attitude but said little. Later she became accusatory in her tone and moderately demeaning toward Gladys.

Gladys's mistrustful and hostile demeanor became exacerbated in response to what she perceived as Ms. H.'s onslaught. When Ms. H. returned from her vacation, Gladys did not come for her appointments. Just as she probably experienced what Ms. H. did when she went on vacation, Gladys disappeared. Attempts by Ms. H. to reach Gladys had no effect.

In order to do successful therapy, the clinician should be able to feel comfortable being the object of a wide range of affects. If she has strong wishes to be consistently loved and admired, she will have to face being overtly rejected time and time again. To keep patients in treatment, the practitioner has to be able to be the recipient, from time to time, of the slings and arrows of the patient's emotions. Being able to be loved is not enough.

FEAR OF BEING AUTHENTIC

One of the serious problems neophyte clinicians inevitably experience is that they begin to lose the spontaneity and authenticity they once owned. Trained to measure their responses carefully, encouraged to listen much and say little, admonished to reveal little about themselves, many clinicians after two or three years of practice can sound more like automatons than the vulnerable and emotional human beings they really are.

Over the years I have observed many caring, enthusiastic, and bright beginners lose their authenticity as they repeatedly and mechanically "learn" to say, "Why do you ask?" "How do you feel?" "It must be hard for you." Like latency children who become frightened of their impulses and develop rigid and punitive superegos, many practitioners can become more preoccupied with technical rules and procedures than with the fears, anxieties, concerns, and responses of their patients. When this occurs, the result might be that the "correct" technique was used but the patient quit!

Just as when an athlete, actor, or virtually any professional is too self-conscious, her performance will become constricted and her audience will respond negatively, the overly self-conscious therapist will not receive very much applause. Rather, her audience is likely to walk out on her.

When the practitioner truly identifies with the patient, really attempts to put herself in his shoes, feels his emotions, and senses his conflicts, she is more likely to be genuine and authentic in her dealings with the patient.

The reason genuineness and authenticity are important therapeutic assets is that patients very much value these qualities (Fine 1982) and are much more inclined to stay in treatment with a therapist who is real than with one who is a mechanical technician.

Isidore, a single man in his early forties, sought treatment with Dr. J., a male psychiatrist in private practice. Isidore wanted treatment because he had severe sexual problems, finding himself sexually impotent on many occasions with the women he desired.

During Isidore's first few months of treatment, while Dr. J. was quiet and listened attentively, Isidore complained about his symptoms and his "sad fate." During the third month of therapy, Dr. J. decided to focus on Isidore's passivity and told him he was frightened of his aggression. Isidore listened to Dr. J.'s interpretations, felt "they were valid," but also told Dr. J. that he was coming across as "cold and distant."

Dr. J. interpreted Isidore's complaints about him as emanating from a wish for an "indulgent parent." Feeling "criticized" and "misunderstood," Isidore left treatment. In effect, he had become impotent with Dr. J.

In his next treatment experience with Dr. K., a woman therapist, Isidore found himself feeling "very understood" when Dr. K. at one point said, "When I put myself in your shoes I feel lost and uncared for." He felt "very given to" when Dr. K. pointed out, "I think you are more of a sexy man than you realize." Dr. K.'s authenticity not only helped Isidore stay in treatment but he felt much more of a man, enough to be consistently potent with women.

One "technique" that I have found helpful when I have tried to formulate what to say to a patient is to ask myself what I would like to hear if I were in the same circumstances that my patient is in. If it does nothing else, it helps me become more of a human being and less of a technician, more a real professional and less a robot. When I feel free to acknowledge that I am a vulnerable human being, I have learned time and again that my patients have an easier time doing the same.

THE THERAPIST'S NEED FOR CONTROL

Many practitioners find it difficult to differentiate between being an authority—which they are—and being authoritarian—which they should not be. Just as a child needs parents who are free to provide structure and ground rules but who also can listen and learn from their children, patients need a similar type of nurturing from their therapists.

It is only in recent years that mental health professionals have been able to grasp the notion that patients can serve as able consultants to us, are capable of giving us sound supervision, and are often correct when they criticize us. I remember learning and gaining a great deal from a 4-year-old male patient, who said to me on more than one occasion, "Dr. Strean, you work too hard, why don't you relax more?" I also recall benefiting much from a teenager who advised, "You talk too much." And, with much warm gratitude, I think often of a woman patient in her forties who was not very familiar with psychotherapeutic parlance but wisely said, "I think they call it 'transference' and you concentrate on it too much."

If the practitioner is unable to listen to patients talk about her vulnerabilities, her idiosyncrasies, and her limitations, she puts a formidable barrier between herself and her patients and indirectly invites them to leave her.

> Leah, a married woman in her mid-fifties, was in treatment with Mr. M., a therapist in private practice. Leah sought treatment because she found herself with much time on her hands and didn't know what to do with herself. Her husband was busy at work and her children were permanently out of the home.
>
> In her sessions with Mr. M., Leah found his constant questioning of her quite irritating and intrusive. After she summoned the necessary courage and told Mr. M. that she found it difficult to answer so many questions in one interview, Mr. M., without realizing it, asked her another question, inquiring, "What is difficult about answering questions?" This activated enormous annoyance in Leah and she angrily admonished, "Take it easy. Let's just chat!"
>
> Again Mr. M. antagonized Leah by asking her, "Why do you want me to take it easy? And why do you want me to just chat with you?" Mr. M.'s stubbornness and need for control eventually "helped" Leah to leave treatment.

In order to help patients stay in treatment and derive benefit from it, the practitioner must let the patient take control from time to time and occasionally take control for a long time. Many of our patients feel so vulnerable that they must always be in control. If the therapist cannot permit this, she may not have a patient any more.

A NEED FOR MUTUAL DEPENDENCY

Anyone who aspires to be a psychotherapist is not only interested in human interaction but also has a strong wish to participate in human relationships. In effect, a therapist, by definition, is *dependent* on her patients in order to make a living. And if she is interested in making a good living, she will usually want her patients to be with her for extended periods of time.

We therapists have not found it easy to acknowledge that we are *more dependent* on other human beings than most people in our society. To carry on our lives we need our patients. And, as we have suggested several times throughout this text, as we go about trying to heal our patients, we are vicariously attempting to heal ourselves as well as our parents, siblings, and significant others (Maroda 1994, Sussman 1992). Consequently, our patients are extremely important people in our lives.

When a therapist, who is by definition a dependent human being, gets together with a patient, who is also a dependent human being, the possibility of a mutually dependent relationship is very strong, if not likely. It is important for the practitioner to assess carefully what she wants from the patient and how gratifying her wishes will help the patient, if at all. We practitioners have often performed splendidly as we help patients get in touch with what they want from us. In addition, we have been of enormous assistance when we could show them what is unrealistic and what is realistic about their desires. However, we have not done a thorough job in educating ourselves in this area so that we can learn some of the same lessons that we try to teach our patients.

Without realizing it, our patients can serve as son or daughter substitutes, as well as substitutes for friends, spouses, lovers, and parents. For those of us who have practiced social work, we could have taken notice of this phenomenon very directly when we made home visits.

Like mature parents who need their children in many ways, we mental health professionals have to be aware of what our wishes are toward our patients, and how we can hurt or help them if we gratify ourselves. As we have already suggested, many of the love-and-be-loved relationships between therapists and patients force the patient's aggression and assertive capacities to go underground. This either leads to premature termination of treatment or creates an ongoing "therapeutic" relationship between patient and therapist that does not foster too much growth in either party.

Very often the advice-giving, environment-manipulating, and supportive therapist is as dependent on her patients as she is on making them dependent on her.

Norman, a man in his mid-forties, was a patient in a treatment center and was being seen by Ms. O., a social worker. Norman came to the center because his son needed treatment, and both Norman and his wife were invited to participate in the treatment. Norman's 9-year-old son, Peter, was having a lot of difficulty in school. He could not feel free to use his own resources and constantly needed help from his teachers and peers. This same helplessness also appeared to be true in Peter's day-to-day activities at home.

As is true in most parent–child situations, Peter's behavior mirrored the behavior of his parents, who were also quite passive and inclined to appear helpless. Consequently, in the therapy situation, Norman constantly sought Ms. O.'s direction and advice. Not realizing that she was doing to Norman what he was doing to Peter, Ms. O. gave Norman advice constantly, visited Peter's school regularly, and in general reinforced Norman's dependency on her.

Because both Peter and Norman were kept very dependent, no improvement took place in either's functioning. After about seven months of treatment, on the advice of a friend, Norman quit treatment and took Peter to another therapist.

Very often, when there is no movement in treatment, the therapist is fostering a mutually dependent relationship between herself and the patient. Although this is initially gratifying to both patient and therapist, it rarely helps the patient mature and frequently leads to early termination of therapy.

THE EROTIC COUNTERTRANSFERENCE

Ever since the formal inception of psychotherapy as a profession, psychotherapists have had major difficulties in monitoring their sexual wishes toward their patients. In Freud's inner circle, Otto Rank turned his patient, Anais Nin, into his mistress. Ernest Jones, Freud's biographer, spent a good part of his career fending off accusations that he sexually molested young patients and had sexual intercourse with older ones. Sandor Ferenczi believed that his patients needed physical comfort; therefore, he openly fondled their breasts and hugged them frequently. Carl Jung had prolonged affairs with several of his patients, including one who became a therapist (Grosskurth 1991).

Sexual activity with patients by the pioneers of psychotherapy has been more than replicated by their followers and contemporaries. In the April 13, 1992, issue of *Newsweek* magazine, it was well documented that a spate of cases involving sexual liaisons between patients and therapists has come to the public's attention in the last decade (Beck 1992). Although at least 10 to 20 percent of those mental health practitioners who have been queried on the subject acknowledge sexual activity with their patients, their numbers are probably higher. Many clinicians, despite being granted anonymity, are frightened to tell the truth because they fear retribution (Gabbard 1989).

In my own research (Strean 1992), I was able to document that most therapists who have sex with their patients are giving to their patients what they secretly wanted from their own therapists (and/or from other parental figures) but were not able to master these wishes. In conducting this research I discovered that most therapists have strong erotic wishes toward many of their patients but often have to handle these wishes by denial, reaction formation, or sadistic behavior.

Even though it is undesirable for therapists to act out their attraction toward their patients, creating a situation that is analogous to incest (Gabbard 1989), it is quite the opposite to have feelings. As Reuben Fine (1982) has stated:

> The more the therapist is able to experience a genuine liking for the patient, the more help he or she will be able to give. Because of the need to keep feelings in check, the [therapist] often takes the path of least resistance, denying them altogether. This creates another problem for the patient, who in addition to feeling rejected for neurotic reasons, is being rejected in reality. The fact that the therapist's rejection is a neurotic defense mechanism to protect him or her against his or her own sexual feelings does not alter the matter; in this way the [therapist] does not differ from other opposite-sex people whom the patient meets. [p. 103]

As psychotherapists have matured, they are more able to acknowledge that, like all humans, they are sexual beings. To deny this reality to our patients is to reinforce their own inhibitions and may be as deleterious as acting out with them. Dr. Harold Searles (1975) averred that, even with very emotionally disturbed women patients, it is crucial to give them the feeling that they are realistically attractive to the therapist. Said Searles:

> Since I began doing psychoanalysis and intensive psychotherapy, I have found, time after time, that in the course of the work with every one of my patients who has progressed to, or very far towards, a thoroughgoing analytic cure, I have experienced romantic and erotic desires to marry, and fantasies of being married to, the patient. [p. 284]

I have found that when a therapist cannot accept her erotic feelings toward the patient and his toward her, one of the favorite defense mechanisms used is to ascribe the patient's desire to his unresolved past.

When Roland, a single man in his early thirties, began to speak of how attractive he found his female therapist to be, Dr. S. initially reacted with mild pleasure. However, as Roland began to describe in detail how he would like to make love to Dr. S., she began to actively interpret to him that he was trying to gratify wishes that he had toward his mother when he was a young boy. Roland protested and said, "Maybe, but I love you and would like you as a lover."

Just as Roland protested when he heard Dr. S.'s interpretations, Dr. S. protested when she heard Roland's remarks. Eventually, Roland gave up and went to another therapist, which may have been what Dr. S. unconsciously wanted.

In his second treatment session with Ms. T., when Roland discussed his erotic wishes toward her, Ms. T. found herself feeling very turned on by him. However, in contrast to Dr. S., she shared with him the fact that if she were not his therapist, she would really enjoy having an affair with him. This heightened Roland's self-esteem as well as his genuine respect for Ms. T.

Treatment was very successful and enabled Roland to move comfortably toward women; eventually he made a successful marriage.

The erotic countertransference, like all countertransference reactions, needs to be accepted as a fact of therapeutic life. The more erotic countertransference reactions are understood by the therapist, the more she can help her patients make substantial and constructive changes.

What we have determined with regard to the erotic countertransference should serve as a guide in coping with countertransference reactions in general. First, we must try our best to accept our wishes and not judge them. Second, we should try to understand why we are experiencing the patient the way we do. Is he trying to induce the feelings we have? If so, why? Finally, the more we can acknowledge the fact that we are always having emotional reactions toward our patients, the more we can help them to feel their feelings and increase their capacity to be loving with others.

CHAPTER EIGHT

THE FINALE:
THE DYNAMICS OF
QUITTING TREATMENT:
CONTRIBUTIONS BY
THERAPIST AND PATIENT

As we move toward the end of our rather prolonged journey, it may be helpful to review some of our major findings. What are the main points that we want to recall from our travels?

Inasmuch as the psychotherapeutic process is always an interactive experience in which two parties actively and continually participate, the premature ending of treatment, like all psychotherapeutic phenomena, should be viewed as a contribution from both parties. Furthermore, while the personalities of both the therapist and patient are the central variables in the therapeutic process, what is crucial in understanding the outcome of the therapy is how these two personalities influence each other (Wolman 1972).

Up until recently those clinicians and scholars who studied the dynamics of the premature ending of treatment have focused most of their attention on the patient's contributions—his dynamics, his resistances, his transferences, and his history. What we discovered many times on our journey is that the therapist's contribution must be seriously considered as well. Her dynamics, her resistances, her transferences, and her history are all being expressed in every therapy session and cannot be overlooked. In addition, it is the *interaction* between the patient's dynamics, transferences, and so forth with the therapist's dynamics, transferences, and so forth that must be continually studied in order to fully understand therapeutic success and failure.

In contrast to the model of the wise and healthy therapist ministering to the unwise and sick patient, we learned from our study that this model misrepresents the therapeutic situation and does not do justice in helping us account for what really occurs in therapy. Each participant in the therapeutic situation has his and her anxieties and pathological dependencies, and each is partially a child with his or her internalized parents (Racker 1968). If the anxieties, pathological dependencies, and internalized parents of the patient and therapist complement and supplement each other, the relationship has a good chance of sustaining itself; if they are not congruent, premature termination of therapy is more likely.

In all interpersonal situations, in order to feel comfortable, the individual attempts to induce his or her role partner to enact roles which will maintain the feeling of comfort (Nelson et al. 1968). In the interpersonal psychotherapeutic situation, this phenomenon, of course, occurs as well. The patient will mobilize changing role patterns of cooperation and resistance that will be designed to influence the therapist to modify her role. And the therapist feels minimally obliged to induce the patient to enact a role because the cooperative effort required of the patient may be felt by him as purely formal and ego-dystonic. Therefore, it can be postulated that therapist and patient alike will try to induce one another to enact the role or roles which each deems necessary to maintain and promote the interpersonal situation (Sandler 1976).

When we conceive of the therapeutic relationship as a transactional field with each of the participants enacting roles and trying to influence the role partner to enact certain roles, we can view premature termination less judgmentally and more objectively. There are no sinners and there are no saints in this transaction. There are no victims and no abusers. Each participant is in constant dynamic interaction with the other, and they are both continually influencing the outcome of the treatment.

A role-set that many therapists prescribe for the patient is to come to all of his sessions regularly and on time, say everything that comes to his mind—fantasies, memories, history, and transference reactions—accept the therapist's interventions with enthusiasm, report therapeutic success frequently, express gratitude warmly and often, and pay the fee regularly. When the patient is unable or unwilling to adapt to this role-set, unless the therapist can empathize with the patient's resistance and understand it well so that the patient feels free to resist and can discuss his resistant attitudes in a safe atmosphere, patient dropout is quite likely.

By the same token, most if not all patients prescribe a role-set for the therapist. A popular one is for her to be very loving, act consistently reassuring, make no demands, offer advice easily and sagely, answer questions well and promptly, offer praise in abundance and frequently, be available between sessions, and charge very little for the services offered. When the therapist is unable or unwilling to fulfill the patient's role requirements, the patient begins to consider leaving treatment. Unless the therapist is able to empathize with the patient's frustrations when he does not receive what he wants and offer something to the patient that is rewarding for him, premature termination is again a realistic possibility.

The therapist's task is a formidable one. If she cannot consistently and appropriately absorb the frustrations that the patient induces when he does not wish to cooperate with the practitioner's expectations, the patient will threaten to depart from therapy. Furthermore, if the practitioner cannot cope with the patient's inevitable disappointments with her and offer constructive understanding in an empathetic manner, premature termination is again a real possibility.

In order to help a patient stay in treatment, the therapist has to deny herself a lot of the gratification that she would normally expect to receive in a nontherapeutic relationship. For example, if the patient pleads for help, the therapist wants to extend herself. If the patient is hostile, the therapist wants to retaliate. If the patient is depressed, the therapist wants to console. If the patient is helpless, the therapist wants to take over. The therapist is frequently tempted to enact roles that only reaffirm the patient's conviction that the world is a horrible place (Kantrowitz 1993).

From the inception of the psychotherapeutic contact, when the first telephone call is initiated, throughout the honeymoon state, on to the first treatment crisis, and until termination, transference and countertransference are always in dynamic interplay with each other, as are resistance and counterresistance. Unless the therapist is very sensitive to these variables and uses them to help the patient feel understood and supported, there is a strong likelihood of a working alliance not developing. Then, the patient's motivation for sustaining treatment becomes progressively weakened.

For a therapeutic alliance to develop, one that will help the patient stay in treatment, the therapist is required to listen a great deal and talk very selectively. Patients resent a "know-it-all" because they feel demeaned and weakened. A therapist who empathetically listens without deluging the patient with interventions, such as constant advice, repeated interpretations, and supportive remarks, is more likely to keep the patient in treatment.

Particularly at the beginning of treatment it is absolutely necessary for the patient to have a quiet, nonintrusive, empathetic therapist who helps the patient tell his story and discharge his feelings. For treatment to be sustained, the patient should be able to feel that he is *not* required to reveal more than he wants to, or accept from the therapist more than he wants to.

As the patient is listened to attentively and is treated with "an unconditional positive regard" (Rogers 1951), he is likely to move into the honeymoon stage of treatment and feel loving feelings toward the practitioner. For the treatment to continue positively, the therapist has to be able to feel comfortable not only with the patient's tender and erotic feelings but with her own as well. When there is an absence of a honeymoon, the therapist is probably finding it difficult to permit loving feelings to emerge from the client and/ or herself.

All honeymoons come to an end! Similar to marriage, as reality intrudes, the role partners begin to realize that their wishes and expectations will not be consistently gratified. In addition, whatever resistances they have about closeness and intimacy become more consciously felt. The first treatment crisis (Fine 1982) is an inevitable occurrence in most therapeutic situations, particularly when the treatment is not short-term. For the treatment to be sustained, the practitioner must face the fact that she is going to be demeaned and devalued, during and, often, after the first treatment crisis. If she cannot weather this storm, she is apt to be destroyed. The therapeutic posture that seems necessary during the first treatment crisis is one where the practitioner listens attentively to the patient's resentments without being defensive, so that the patient will be enabled to face the inevitable disappointments, frustrations, and dissatisfactions that therapy always induces. Furthermore, if the patient has realistic criticisms to offer the practitioner about herself, it is often helpful to the therapeutic process if she can acknowledge some of them.

Many patients, if not most, tend to believe that they are the victims of bad circumstances. If only they had a better spouse, a better boss, or a better job, they are positive they would be better off! And if they do not complain about their current reality, they care about their past reality. Although it is important to give the patient plenty of time and space to vent his miseries, it is always important for the practitioner to keep in mind that all chronic complaints are unconscious wishes (Strean 1994). The husband who constantly avers that his wife is "a cold, sexless bitch" unconsciously wants such a wife—a warm, sexy, responsive wife would threaten him too much. Similarly, the wife who complains constantly that her husband is "a weak, passive jerk" wants such a man. A strong, active man would upset her too much.

One of the best ways to help the patient gain some understanding and mastery of his difficult marriage (or parent–child relationship, conflict with the boss, or any other current reality) is for the therapist not to take sides in the marital conflict or in any other of the patient's interpersonal conflicts. If the therapist can remain neutral but empathetic, warm but not indulgent, the patient begins to experience the therapist the same way he experiences his spouse, boss, or child. Then when he notes that he perceives many people the same way, and adds the therapist to his list, he begins to realize that he has a major role in his own interpersonal difficulties. Slowly it dawns on the patient that he is the editor-in-chief of his own interpersonal scripts, and then he is more likely to stay in treatment and try to understand what he does to make his life less fulfilling than it can be.

As the therapist allows transference reactions to be expressed by the patient and focuses on resistive phenomena such as lateness, absences, and nonpayment of fees as interpersonal events that transpire between patient and therapist, the patient slowly begins to diminish his hatred and becomes more loving. He is able to do this because the therapist accepts him as he is and wants nothing much other than to understand him. This attitude helps make the patient feel loved and encourages him to stay in treatment.

One of the most valuable findings of our study is the tremendous role and power of countertransference (Maroda 1994). If the therapist is able to see how she is more similar to the patient than different, realizes that she suffers from many of the same conflicts that the patient does, and tries to gain some mastery over her countertransference issues, the continuation of the therapy is much more assured.

REFERENCES

Abend, S. (1982). Serious illness in the analyst: countertransference considerations. *Journal of the American Psychoanalytic Association* 30:365–379.

———— (1989). Countertransference and psychoanalytic technique. *Psychoanalytic Quarterly* 58:374–395.

Ackerman, N. (1958). *The Psychodynamics of Family Life.* New York: Basic Books.

Barchilon, J. (1958). On countertransference cures. *Journal of the American Psychoanalytic Association* 6:222–236.

Beck, M. (1992). Sex and psychotherapy. *Newsweek,* April 13, pp. 53–57.

Bergmann, M. (1987). *The Anatomy of Loving.* New York: Columbia University Press.

Bernstein, A. (1972). The fear of compassion. In *Success and Failure in Psychoanalysis and Psychotherapy,* ed. B. Wolman, pp. 160–176. New York: Macmillan.

Blanck, G., and Blanck, R. (1974). *Ego Psychology. Theory and Practice.* New York: Columbia University Press.

Boesky, D. (1990). The psychoanalytic process and its components. *Psychoanalytic Quarterly* 59:550–584.

Brenner, C. (1976). *Psychoanalytic Technique and Psychic Conflict.* New York: International Universities Press.

——— (1985). Countertransference as compromise formation. *Psychoanalytic Quarterly* 54:155–163.

Chessick, R. (1971). *Why Psychotherapists Fail.* New York: Jason Aronson.

Consolini, G. (1997). Self-analysis and resistance to self-analysis of countertransference. *Journal of Analytic Social Work* 4(1): 61–82.

Erikson, E. (1950). *Childhood and Society.* New York: Norton.

Feldman, Y. (1958). A casework approach toward understanding parents of emotionally disturbed children. *Social Work* 3:23–29.

Fenichel, O. (1945). *The Psychoanalytic Theory of Neurosis.* New York: Norton.

Fine, R. (1968). Interpretation: the patient's response. In *Use of Interpretation in Treatment: Technique and Art*, ed. E. Hammer, pp. 110–120. New York: Grune & Stratton.

——— (1982). *The Healing of the Mind,* 2nd ed. New York: Free Press.

——— (1985). *The Meaning of Love in Human Experience.* New York: Wiley.

Finell, J. (1985). Narcissistic problems in analysts. *International Journal of Psycho-Analysis* 66:433–445.

——— (1997). *Mind–Body Problems: Psychotherapy with Psychosomatic Disorders.* Northvale, NJ: Jason Aronson.

Freeman, L. (1989). *The Beloved Prison.* New York: St. Martin's.

Freud, A. (1946). *Ego and the Mechanisms of Defense.* New York: International Universities Press.

Freud, S. (1904). Freud's psychoanalytic procedure. *Standard Edition* 7:249–256.

———— (1905). Three essays on the theory of sexuality. *Standard Edition* 7:125–248.

———— (1910). The future prospects of psychoanalytic therapy. *Standard Edition* 11:139–151.

———— (1912). The dynamics of transference. *Standard Edition* 12:97–108.

———— (1923). The ego and the id. *Standard Edition* 19:1–66.

———— (1926). Inhibitions, symptoms, and anxiety. *Standard Edition* 20:77–174.

———— (1938). *The Basic Writings of Sigmund Freud*. New York: Random House.

———— (1939). An outline of psychoanalysis. *Standard Edition* 23:139–251.

Gabbard, G. (1989). *Sexual Exploitation in Professional Relationships*. Washington, DC: American Psychiatric Press.

———— (1996). *Love and Hate in the Analytic Setting*. Northvale, NJ: Jason Aronson.

Glover, E. (1955). *The Technique of Psychoanalysis*. New York: International Universities Press.

Goldstein, E. (1997). To tell or not to tell: the disclosure of events in the therapist's life to the patient. *Clinical Social Work Journal* 25(4):41–59.

Greenson, R. (1967). *The Technique and Practice of Psychoanalysis*. New York: International Universities Press.

Grosskurth, P. (1991). *The Secret Ring*. New York: Addison-Wesley.

Hall, C., and Lindzey, G. (1957). *Theories of Personality*. New York: Wiley.

Hamilton, G. (1951). *Theory and Practice of Social Casework*. New York: Columbia University Press.

Hirsch, I. (1980). Authoritarian aspects of the psychoanalytic relationship. *Review of Existential Psychology and Psychiatry* 17:105–133.

Jacobs, T. (1986). On countertransference enactments. *Journal of the American Psychoanalytic Association* 43:289–307.

Kadushin, A. (1997). *The Social Work Interview,* 4th ed. New York: Columbia University Press.

Kantrowitz, J. (1993). Impasses in psychoanalysis: overcoming resistances in situations of stalemate. *Journal of the American Psychoanalytic Association* 41(4):1021–1050.

Kardiner, A. (1945). *The Psychological Frontiers of Society.* New York: Columbia University Press.

Kernberg, O. (1965). Notes on countertransference. *Journal of the American Psychoanalytic Association* 13:38–56.

——— (1995). *Love Relations: Normality and Pathology.* New Haven, CT: Yale University Press.

Langs, R. (1973). *The Technique of Psychoanalytic Psychotherapy,* vol. 1. Northvale, NJ: Jason Aronson.

——— (1975). The patient's unconscious perception of the therapist's errors. In *Tactics and Techniques in Psychoanalytic Therapy,* vol. II, ed. P. Giovacchini, pp. 230–250. New York: Jason Aronson.

——— (1976). *The Bi-Personal Field.* New York: Jason Aronson.

Lewin, R. (1996). *Compassion: The Core Value That Animates Psychotherapy.* Northvale, NJ: Jason Aronson.

Love, S. and Mayer, H. (1970). Going along with defenses in resistive families. In *New Approaches in Child Guidance,* ed. H. Strean, pp. 124–133. Metuchen, NJ: Scarecrow Press.

Maroda, K. (1994). *The Power of Countertransference.* Northvale, NJ: Jason Aronson.

McDougall, J. (1989). *Theatres of the Body.* New York: Norton.

Nelson, M., Nelson, B., Sherman, M., and Strean, H. (1968). *Roles and Paradigms in Psychotherapy.* New York: Grune & Stratton.

Noble, D., and Hamilton, A. (1983). Coping and complying: a challenge in health care. *Social Work* 28(6):462–466.

Offit, A. (1995). *The Sexual Self.* Northvale, NJ: Jason Aronson.

Racker, H. (1968). *Transference and Countertransference.* New York: International Universities Press.

———— (1972). The meanings and uses of countertransference. *Psychoanalytic Quarterly* 41:487–506.

Raines, J. (1996). Self-disclosure in clinical social work. *Clinical Social Work Journal* 24(4):351–377.

Reich, A. (1951). On countertransference. In *Annie Reich: Psychoanalytic Contributions,* ed. A. Reich, pp. 136–154. New York: International Universities Press.

Reik, T. (1941). *Masochism in Modern Man.* New York: Grove Press.

Renik, O. (1993). Analytic interaction: conceptualizing technique in light of the analyst's irreducible subjectivity. *Psychoanalytic Quarterly* 62:553–571.

Ripple, L., Alexander, E., and Polemis, B. (1964). *Motivation, Capacity and Opportunity.* Chicago: University of Chicago Press.

Rogers, C. (1951). *Client-Centered Therapy.* Boston: Houghton Mifflin.

Sandler, J. (1976). Countertransference and role responsiveness. *International Review of Psycho-Analysis* 3:43–48.

Sandler, J., Dare, C., and Holder, A. (1973). *The Patient and the Analyst: The Basics of the Psychoanalytic Process.* New York: International Universities Press.

Schafer, R. (1995). Aloneness in the countertransference. *Psychoanalytic Quarterly* 64(3):496–516.

Searles, H. (1975). The patient as therapist to his analyst. In *Tactics and Techniques in Psychoanalytic Therapy,* vol. II, ed. P. Giovacchini, pp. 95–151. New York: Jason Aronson.

———— (1979). *Countertransference and Related Subjects.* New York: International Universities Press.

Sherman, M. (1966). *Psychoanalysis in America: Historical Perspectives.* Springfield, IL: Charles C Thomas.

Slakter, E. (1987). *Countertransference.* Northvale, NJ: Jason Aronson.

Sternbach, O. (1947). Arrested ego development and its treatment in conduct disorders and neuroses of childhood. *Nervous Child* 6:306–317.

Strean, H. (1970). The use of the patient as consultant. In *New Approaches in Child Guidance,* ed. H. Strean, pp. 53–63. Metuchen, NJ: Scarecrow Press.

———— (1976). Some psychodynamics in referring patients for psychotherapy. In *Crucial Issues in Psychotherapy,* ed. H. Strean, pp. 130–139. Metuchen, NJ: Scarecrow Press.

———— (1978). *Clinical Social Work.* New York: Free Press.

———— (1980). *The Extramarital Affair.* New York: Free Press.

———— (1983). *The Sexual Dimension.* New York: Free Press.

———— (1986). Why therapists lose clients. *Journal of Independent Social Work* 1:7–17.

———— (1990). *Resolving Resistances in Psychotherapy.* New York: Brunner/Mazel.

———— (1991). *Behind the Couch.* New York: Continuum.

———— (1992). *Therapists Who Have Sex with Their Patients: Treatment and Recovery.* New York: Brunner/Mazel.

———— (1993). *Resolving Counterresistances in Psychotherapy.* New York: Brunner/Mazel.

———— (1994). *Essentials of Psychoanalysis.* New York: Brunner/Mazel.

———— (1995a). *Psychotherapy with the Unattached.* Northvale, NJ: Jason Aronson.

——— (1995b). Countertransference and theoretical predilections as observed in some psychoanalytic candidates. *Canadian Journal of Psychoanalysis* 3(1):105–124.

——— (1996a). *Resolving Marital Conflicts*. Northvale, NJ: Jason Aronson.

——— (1996b). *Mending the Broken Heart: A Psychological Perspective on Preventing and Treating Heart Disease*. Northvale, NJ: Jason Aronson.

——— (1998). *When Nothing Else Works: Innovative Interventions with Intractable Individuals*. Northvale, NJ: Jason Aronson.

Strean, H., and Freeman, L. (1992). *Why People Fail*. Tarrytown, NY: Wynwood Press.

Sullivan, H. (1953). *The Interpersonal Theory of Psychiatry*. New York: Norton.

Sussman, M. (1992). *A Curious Calling: Unconscious Motivations for Practicing Psychotherapy*. Northvale, NJ: Jason Aronson.

Tarachow, S. (1963). *An Introduction to Psychotherapy*. New York: International Universities Press.

Wolman, B. (1972). *Success and Failure in Psychoanalysis and Psychotherapy*. New York: Macmillan.

INDEX